RCR

D1085362

THE
BED REST
SURVIVAL
GUIDE

THE
BED REST
SURVIVAL
GUIDE

BARBARA EDELSTON PETERSON

Foreword by Hallie Beacham, M.D., M.P.H.

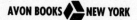
AVON BOOKS ◆ NEW YORK

Note: Some of the accounts in Chapter 7 are composites of more than one person's experience. The names and identifying characteristics of these people have been altered to protect their privacy.

AVON BOOKS, INC.
1350 Avenue of the Americas
New York, New York 10019

Copyright © 1998 by Barbara Edelston Peterson
Foreword © 1998 by Hallie Beacham, M.D.,M.P.H.
Front cover illustration by Julie Johnson
Published by arrangement with the author
Visit our website at **http://www.AvonBooks.com**
ISBN: 0-380-79506-X

Library of Congress Cataloging in Publication Data:
Peterson, Barbara Edelston.
The bedrest survival guide / by Barbara Edelston Peterson.
p. cm.
1. Bed rest—Psychological aspects. 2. Pregnancy—
Complications—Prevention. 3. Adjustment (Psychology)—
Popular works. I. Title.
RG572.P39 1998   98-9587
615.5—dc21   CIP

First Avon Books Trade Printing: June 1998

AVON TRADEMARK REG. U.S. PAT. OFF. AND IN OTHER COUNTRIES, MARCA
REGISTRADA, HECHO EN U.S.A.

Printed in the U.S.A.

QPM 10 9 8 7 6 5 4 3 2 1

Dedicated in love to Dick, Hilary, and Foreste.

Contents

FOREWORD
1

INTRODUCTION
3

CHAPTER ONE
Finding Inspiration
7

CHAPTER TWO
Immediate Preparation
16

CHAPTER THREE
Creating a Routine
29

CHAPTER FOUR
Bedside Entertainment and Personal Projects
39

CHAPTER FIVE
Smart and Savory Picnics
63

CHAPTER SIX
Sexuality and Bed Rest
79

CHAPTER SEVEN
You're Not Alone
85

APPENDIX A
Affirmations
128

APPENDIX B
Self-help Bibliography
132

APPENDIX C
Who's Who at the Doctor's Office
134

APPENDIX D
Important Phone Numbers
138

APPENDIX E
Home Services and Supply Sources
158

ACKNOWLEDGMENTS
163

Foreword

by Hallie Beacham, M.D., M.P.H.

Every year, legions of patients are prescribed bed rest as part of a treatment regimen. Many of these prescriptions are for obstetrical patients, orthopedic patients, accident victims, and ophthalmic patients. When prescribed for these persons, bed rest becomes as important as any potion or pill.

Bed rest, however, is more intangible than medication, and is invariably prescribed for a patient who is least apt to find this form of therapy welcome news. This is especially true for the pregnant patient who is being treated for preterm labor.

As a physician I routinely describe to patients the potential side effects of medications. I indicate how often the medications should be taken. This information is then reinforced by the pharmacist, who provides labels highlighting the most significant side effects. As an obstetrician, when I first began to prescribe bed rest as a part of a regimen to control preterm labor, it seemed so simple and straightforward. Medical side effects might be blood clots in the legs, as a result of prolonged inactivity of the legs and the resultant decrease in blood flow; constipation could be an issue. What I did not initially anticipate were some of the other consequences of prescribing bed rest.

In the not-too-distant past, the vast majority of patients treated with bed rest were confined to hospitals for a much more significant portion of their illness. That meant nurses and occupational therapists and any number of other paraprofessionals could observe any physical and psychological problems the patient developed and minister to them.

Now, with patients spending far less time in hospitals and families dependent on two incomes, the fallout from the bed rest prescription frequently rests squarely on the shoulders of the "infirm"! For obstetrical patients, inactivity is frequently thrust on an unwilling recipient who is excited about her pregnancy but who has just been informed of an immense disruption in her life. She's frightened about the possible outcome of her pregnancy. At this time the mother often isn't considering her own comfort but rather the medical threat to her baby, and, as a result, she doesn't ask or retain important information about her prescribed bed rest. Being at home—not in a hospital where she might seek continual paraprofessional input—has added to the problems experienced by bed rest patients.

I began to learn of these concerns as patients returned for their visits and shared their experiences with me. Patients told me they were now working ONLY four hours a day, not eight, or that they were home but they were using the stairs seven times a day. Since then, I've learned to be very specific in defining "bed rest." The written word is an invaluable adjunct to instruction given in the office.

Having experienced bed rest herself, Barbara Edelston Peterson found she wanted solutions to myriad issues presented by her confinement. As a result, she's produced a comprehensive guide to help the new bed rest patient negotiate this experience in the most tolerable fashion possible. In this book, she shares her lessons and invaluable words for medical professionals and any new patient prescribed bed rest.

Introduction

The Bed Rest Survival Guide is the first personal handbook offering inspirational and practical guidance for bedridden people in search of a way to make the most of their time in bed. It is for individuals confined to bed rest while healing a curable medical problem. This book would not be appropriate for people with chronic illness or for those elderly who spend their remaining days in bed.

The number of people prescribed temporary bed rest is staggering. The largest single group is pregnant women. Five million women each year have viable pregnancies and 20 percent of them require bed rest. **This means a potential one million women need this book, every year.** Another seven million people, men and women, are prescribed bed rest to treat a variety of other problems, including: neck, back, hip, and head pain and injury; sciatica; blood-volume regulation; arthritis; cardiovascular dysfunction; and bone degeneration.

So why did I write this book?

This kind of resource would have been *invaluable* to me when I had to go on bed rest in the winter of 1989. Through trial and error, my husband and I groped our way through a three-month-long journey. We had absolutely no experience with anything like bed rest. At the time, we were busy professionals and avid cyclists and skiers with a full social life. When we were suddenly confronted by this unexpected circumstance, we received no guidance whatsoever. We were truly "bed rest pioneers" in our search to find comfort and make the most out of a totally unexpected and unfamiliar situation. We found ourselves awed by our makeshift creations and positive experiences. Toward the end of the "term," I knew I would have to tell my story to inspire and motivate others trying to endure the bed rest experience.

The Bed Rest Survival Guide is neither medical nor technical in nature. It is an instructive and inspirational guide for making the most of your time in bed. I've focused on providing you with emotional encouragement, practical suggestions, creative ideas, and spiritual guidance.

I envision you keeping this book at arm's reach. My hope is that you will use it like you would an office "daytimer." Whether you've used one or not, you may find that *The Bed Rest Survival Guide* becomes your "daytimer" *and* "nighttimer"! I recommend that you read the first two chapters immediately because my suggestions provide exactly what you'll need for basic bed rest survival. Then, once you are settled, the other chapters will reveal additional important alternatives for your continued comfort on bed rest. I hope that this book becomes your personal companion and provides you with positive reinforcement for every hour of every day.

Staying still and in bed for more than one night's sleep is a challenge to anyone's basic nature. Responding to a prognosis that requires the bed rest prescription demands an entirely different level of attention and acceptance. My experience stemmed from the desire to see a healthy firstborn child. Your situation may be similar or of a completely different nature. However, each patient is forced to consider the same dilemma: how am I going to endure the daunting prospect of enforced stillness? And although the immediate reaction to lying still for an undetermined period of time is disconcerting, I can assure you it is not the most difficult moment of bed rest.

Before too long, the bedridden patient discovers it is the moments ahead—the many moments of every day, every week, and every month—that require a commitment to living in a completely different manner than accustomed.

Before I was prescribed bed rest, my life was overflowing with commitments. I had a full-time marketing job, daily athletics, a new marriage, and a busy social schedule. After my doctor ordered bed rest, I felt like I was being sentenced to prison. There was little direction, support, or advice from the medical staff, only the strict words to eliminate any temptation for detours between the bed and the bathroom. What was I supposed to do?

Since my own time on bed rest, I've discovered my situation was not unique. Most people are at a total loss for what to do—not only on a practical level but on a deeply personal level. With so little help available, *The Bed Rest Survival Guide* is bound to make a difference—not only for you, but for your families and friends, and for patient care in general.

In addition to its being a practical guide, I have developed this book to encourage people to truly benefit from this experience. Whether you are in bed many weeks or many months, the experience presents an ongoing challenge, but it can be well managed with sensitivity and a supportive home-care system. My own inventions, as well as ingenious ideas from others, fill the book with commonsense solutions and creative ideas. Most of the book's practical and creative elements, as well as the information in the appendices, provide valuable resources for enjoying life more fully on bed rest.

As a bed rest veteran, I deeply believe that everyone's experience during bed rest can be a gift and not a curse. After reading this book, I hope that you will agree that your greatest lesson from bed rest is similar to what I discovered, that our highs in life come not from doing any single thing, but from the inner strength we feel when we successfully face a challenge and overcome the obstacles.

CHAPTER ONE

Finding Inspiration

Suddenly a Change in Life

Under normal circumstances when we're tired and need rest, the bed is seductively warm and peaceful. Once a doctor instructs us to remain in bed for an undetermined period of time, however, our former haven represents only confinement and anxiety.

At twenty-four weeks gestation with my first pregnancy, I went into preterm labor and was unexpectedly prescribed bed rest. At the time, the prospect of this confinement was something I knew nothing about.

I remember the first moments after being told I would have to stay completely still. My first response was to acknowledge my doctor, and without emotion, shake my head, and say, "OK, that's fine."

My world then changed.

There are as many reactions to such an extreme change in lifestyle as there are approaches to survival. For me, confinement triggered reactions of resistance, disappointment, fear, and anger. I felt empty. The initial void threatened my identity and dramatically upset my sense of personal balance. Normally, I come and go at a very fast pace, and I'm very independent. With this new mandate, I was left to figure out how to proceed: what would be the next-best strategy for living?

A dynamically busy lifestyle had unexpectedly changed to one of enforced stillness.

Your world may also feel as though it has just collapsed—you may be weakened by feelings that rapidly ping-pong among fear, disbelief, amazement, and sheer numbness.

I can remember when the doctor left the hospital room after telling me I must remain in bed until possibly the end of my pregnancy term. As the door closed behind her, I burst into tears. I was scared. I felt like everything in my life had just blacked out. My mind began racing with fears about the health of my baby, my career, and my dedication to staying in shape.

How would my husband do everything? We certainly couldn't afford help. What would our life be like now? How long would it be until I would be free to feel the sun or breathe fresh air again? I was filled with endless concerns about how bed rest would affect every aspect of my life.

I thought bed rest meant a living death. But slowly, a new reality unfolded. I began to consider the possibilities: how could I accomplish the things I love to do, and *had* to do, while in bed?

I realized that if I were to survive another day, I would have to open my mind, shift my heart, and focus my energy. As overwhelming as all of this was, I felt there was no choice but to reorient myself to this new world of stillness.

From somewhere within, I noticed an inner voice coaching me to let go of what I knew to be normal and begin accepting what temporarily lay before me. I began to think more openly and found myself considering in positive terms the fact that life rarely offers this kind of respite from the chaos of everyday life. Bed rest can eventually become an experience that is very peaceful. It can also become a place in your life where innovation and resourcefulness thrive. And although the abundance of free time can be hard at first, it was something I grew to treasure. As the days passed, I began to feel more free. A new lifestyle emerged, as did new priorities. I wanted more than anything to ensure the health of both my baby and myself. I figured out how to be still and follow the rules, and yet enjoy a very active life.

I had the advantages of an optimistic nature and strong will-power. They helped buoy me through the days, weeks, and months ahead.

Psychologist Roberto Assagioli wrote specifically about the powers of the will. He once said, "The discovery of the will in oneself, and even more the realization that the self and the will are intimately connected, may come as a real revelation which can change, often radically, a person's self-awareness and his whole attitude toward himself, other people and the world."

In many areas of our lives, we consciously use willpower. For dieting, exercising, or finishing a job we rely on willpower. In my bed rest experience, I found that in reaching deep within to find strength and will, I was able to move beyond the fear and sadness that might have otherwise consumed me. I started by facing my feelings, validating them, and then shifting my focus from fear and self-pity to making plans and taking action.

I had the will—now I had to find the way.

In your efforts to manage the challenge, it may be helpful to use willpower in seeing the situation from another vantage point. We all know the bed has qualities that normally soothe the body, soul, and mind. Why not use this perspective to your advantage? I discovered that in seeing my bed as a protective nest, it became a special place, where I felt well nurtured. In its safety, I found comfort, inner strength, and, eventually, a new kind of happiness.

Think of the possibilities. Summon your will. There *is* a way for you, too.

The Journey Begins with Acceptance

Finding a balance between activity and quietude is what I have defined as the natural reality for bed rest. Opening oneself to the acceptance process while minimizing expectations is key to feeling genuinely calm in this new reality. I found that as soon as I emptied my mind of pre–bed rest standards and expectations, I no longer felt so aimless. I began to feel more peaceful. The physical limitations felt less threatening. I was able to accept more easily the parameters of my new lifestyle.

This does not have to be a time to feel deprived or desperate—or a time to feel passive or defeated. Bed rest can be a wholesome opportunity for regeneration and healing. It is a quiet time. It is also a time for as much activity as one would naturally be inclined toward, simply in a different context.

I found it very helpful to learn everything there was to know about my specific condition. With more knowledge of the medical issues, I felt my need for control ease. The information you receive about your specific medical condition will empower you to move beyond the endless questions.

In my survey of people who have experienced bed rest for various reasons, the majority of them agree that the burden eventually becomes a tolerable challenge. In most cases, bed rest was later considered one of life's most memorable experiences. Whether a pregnancy complication, a back injury, a degenerative hip, or a viral disability, the temporary nature of this solution is a small price to pay for the results of successful healing.

One will discover how quickly the mind surrenders its initial rejection and finds acceptance in the refuge of bed rest.

An old Chinese saying inspired me from the beginning of my time on bed rest. "An inch of time is an inch of gold: Treasure it. Appreciate its fleeting nature; misplaced gold is easily found, misspent time is lost forever." It helped me to accept bed rest as a natural part of life's expression—a bump along the path. A bump that can offer valuable lessons.

Maintaining a good life on bed rest is easier when mental energy is used in a positive and productive way. Let's face it, bed rest is difficult for everyone, but if you are a low-key individual who is content to rest, bed rest might be less of an effort. If you are a high-energy type, chances are you'll find that you're just as lively, only in a different way.

I began to feel hopeful.

Intellectually, you may understand the influence of positive and negative thoughts. Now, you can experience their real effects. On bed rest, a negative attitude will produce a lonely, boring, painful experience.

I experienced firsthand how a positive attitude improved my health as well as ensured a fruitful, creative, dynamic adventure that in turn delivered the full life on bed rest which I originally thought impossible.

Once I began focusing on what I *could* do rather than the limitations imposed by bed rest, the experience changed for me. I got back the work via the telephone. I explored activities that excited me. I felt my energy return. It began to sink in. Enforced stillness was the chance of a lifetime to pursue the things I'd always wanted to but never had the time for.

Whether it be learning a new language, reading every volume on a particular subject matter, or finishing the family photo albums, the opportunity is yours. With a positive outlook, the will to heal, and a curious mind, you can easily find inspiration in the bed rest reality.

In life, when you reach beyond the status quo and do what you love, you produce a positive experience. On bed rest, you can find creative ways to use the time which will not only enhance your experience but will provide you with energy for optimal healing.

Letting go and accepting bed rest can be an emotional struggle. Naturally, there will be times of frustration and impatience.

I had a good cry every other day, but I was rarely left feeling sad.

Emotions help release energy and support the process of letting go and moving on. Confident thinking in conjunction with the use of affirmations helps give life to the ever-important positive attitude toward healing. Appendix A in the back of this book will guide you through effective use of affirmations.

Norman Cousins wrote, "The greatest force in the human body is the natural drive of the body to heal itself—but that force is not independent of the belief system, which can translate expectations into physiological change. Nothing is more wondrous about the fifteen billion neurons in the human brain than their ability to convert thoughts, hopes, ideas, and attitudes into chemical substances. Everything begins, therefore, with belief. What we believe is the most powerful option of all."

Believe in yourself. You can do it!

On bed rest, we are people challenged by physical stipulations that require psychological adaptation.

Before I went on bed rest, I was dependent on physical activity as a release from my busy lifestyle. Competition played a prominent role in my life. A month before I was pregnant, I swam in a relay across Lake Tahoe. Six months later I would be in bed for three months.

The choice was presented—to respond by lamenting or by acceptance. I pondered over the famous serenity prayer that I had not understood as well as I do now, "God grant me the serenity to accept the things I cannot change, the courage to change the things I can, and the wisdom to know the difference."

Having courage and wisdom came through in the form of reaching out to family and friends for help. The love and support I received in return gave me a sense of purpose at a time when I felt so vulnerable. I grew to believe that I would make it through this epic adventure.

Bed Rest as Teacher

In our culture, illness and physical disabilities are often viewed as problems that occur from outside us. The inconvenient healing process is usually facilitated by the use of medication. What I learned by accepting and moving beyond this standard is that the process can be a marvelous teacher.

The bed rest experience encouraged me to look at patterns throughout my life, and to see that all of life is an ever-changing process.

Often, the unexpected becomes reality.

I realized that no matter who you are or how you live, there will *always* be twists and turns along the path of life that require adaptation.

Bed rest can make you realize your ability to change your life when you need to—to drive down a new road and not feel lost. Whether we intend the adventurous route for the sake of challenge or we are caught by the unexpected, respect for change and a willingness to make adjustments is the way toward graceful living.

When I reflect on times of struggle in my life, I see striking similarities between the process of adapting to the experience of bed rest and other transitional events. When it was the first day at a different school or starting a new job, each experience required an adjustment that included some discomfort. Each prompted resistance to adapting to new conditions. Each experience eventually led to acceptance, with a commitment to rise above the fear and make the most of the situation.

Acceptance opens up potential channels for new skills. And when we see our ability to overcome our fears, we are rewarded with a deeper confidence and an inner calm.

I had a life-altering experience at age sixteen. I joined a mountaineering expedition that ventured into the heart of Wyoming's Wind River Mountains.

As the youngest in a large group, I found myself physically exhausted and psychologically overwhelmed. Climbing above 11,000 feet for two of the six weeks, scaling by rope and ice ax, eating only essential food to survive, and being stranded one night atop the highest point in Wyoming in the midst of an electrical storm, tested every cell of my being.

I never thought I would make it, but I did.

Like the adventure of bed rest, this event could have been a horror had there not been the common lesson of learning strength from weakness. I now refer to this experience as the adventure of my life. (And by the way, I now refer to bed rest as the time of my life!)

Each experience called for its own balanced acceptance of the present—good or bad. Each helped me better understand life's intricate mechanics. Each was an illustrative example that the healer was within.

The lesson: challenges offer opportunities to develop new skills—physical and emotional.

In my determination to find meaningful activity in bed, I discovered personal resources I never knew existed. Whether learning to sew, writing a poem, or manifesting a speedy recovery, I learned how to depend on myself for stimulation rather than the outside world.

Nobody can make it work but you. We are what we believe we can be!

The experience also taught me about healing. Some pain is inevitable. Suffering is optional.

Sometimes crisis teaches self-love and compassion. My time on bed rest provided me with a more compassionate perspective on those who have mobility problems. It also allowed me to care for myself in a way that felt loving, not selfish.

One of the most valuable lessons of bed rest may be in letting go of the need to be in control. Another lesson might be learning how to receive and accept whatever someone else has to offer and letting them take more control. Accepting help graciously is an art equal to giving.

The experience gave me another way of looking at life while identifying the value of what is meaningful. The bed rest experience is the ultimate lesson in patience. Hours, days, and weeks of enforced stillness teach resourcefulness and flexibility in the face of time.

Now, whenever I am in a situation that requires waiting for extended periods of time without a book, newspaper, or some other source of entertainment, I reflect back on the patience of being bedridden for three months. That comparison eases whatever tension I feel.

Patience was the beginning of a process toward inner peace for me. As I remained bedridden, acknowledging my feelings and learning to accept myself in that situation became crucial, not only for enhancing physical healing but for living peacefully.

Whether you're temporarily on bed rest or not, the path to

peace is the same: finding a way to *be yourself,* holding a reverence for life, and doing what makes you feel special and well nurtured.

Change in all of us evolves slowly, but finding inner peace is a way to bring grace and steadiness to everything life presents.

CHAPTER TWO

Immediate preparation

*H*umans are energy systems, whether enduring bed rest or pursuing normal daily functions. Every moment of every day, we manage personal energy: we wake up with it, we direct it, we store it, we process it. We are very much in control of how our energy gets used and where it is focused. For every individual, the way energy is spent determines the integrity and quality of personal life.

Although bed rest dictates a physically slower-paced existence, it does not have to lower your energy level or quality of life. Bed rest actually demands a lot of energy with a new focus on managing a new lifestyle. This chapter offers suggestions for ways to prosper while bedridden. I believe the secret to success is developing and maintaining a positive belief system that focuses on a successful end result. With this kind of perspective you can discover the ability to manage life well and actually to enjoy the gift of time while on bed rest.

THE ESSENTIAL CHECKLIST

- *Call all important people in your life:* family, colleagues, friends, and local community members (school, synagogue or church, book club, etc.) to let them know you are on bed rest. You do not want to be isolated, and you will need all the support and help you can get.

- *Call your insurance carrier.* They will need to know the details of your temporary disability. Important: Inquire about home service coverage: home care, physical therapy (try to cover massage under this category), medical supplies (rentals and purchases), etc. If you are pregnant, you may want to inquire about coverage in the event of complications during delivery (cesarean section) or extra care if your baby is born prematurely.

- *File for disability insurance.* Call your local Employment Development Department and have the papers sent to your home. Expect the instructions to be simple and straightforward. You may need your employer's signature, which you can obtain by mail if no one from Human Resources can make a personal visit.

- *Arrange for access to your home.* Put an extra key somewhere outside so that select people can get into your home. Expect to receive visits and help from a variety of different people. (You are in control of this, always. Be clear when you do *not* want someone to visit. State directly that for now it would be uncomfortable to have a visit, and you would appreciate their honoring your feelings at this time. Example: After one visit from my boss, a great guy but very hyper, I had to request we continue to work over the telephone rather than face-to-face. His "enthusiasm" caused an increase in contractions.)
  Important: Make sure the key is returned every time!

- *Supplies that provide immediate comfort:* (see detailed list in "The Accessorized Bed" section)

- ❏ Cordless telephone
- ❏ Good mattress
- ❏ Small cooler to place on the bed
- ❏ Large plastic cup with straw or a tall cup with built-in straw
- ❏ Lightweight cot for mobility

🌀 *Set up communication.* Each family member or care provider should carry a beeper, so there's never a chance, in case of an emergency, you're out of touch.

🌀 *Child-proof your surroundings!* When you are confined, this is an ideal time for children to get into things.

🌀 *Cash on hand.* You will want to reimburse people who pick things up for you, run errands, etc. It will help you feel more comfortable receiving the favors. *Important: Do not give anyone a blank check or your ATM card unless it's your partner, a very close relative or friend.*

🌀 *Bedside table.* This will be the anchor for your ship! It will hold all of your tools for survival. (See "The Accessorized Bed" section for more detail.)

🌀 *Gather important phone numbers:* doctors, nurses, hospitals, insurance, work, family, friends—the phone is your link to the outside world! Use the phone book in the back of your *Bed Rest Survival Guide.* It will help you feel organized. Have your own address book at arm's reach.

🌀 *Deciding who might live in and help:* whether a relative or friend, consider what you need right now and who might best fit in to your household situation. The ideal live-in person might be someone who has most of the following traits:

—is comfortable taking over responsibilities
—is self-entertaining
—respects your values and style
—understands your need for quiet time, private time
—supports your relationship
—is a positive individual and emotionally stable

☙ *Hire housekeeping* if you can afford it. Ideally, this person should have a car to do errands outside of the home, prepare meals, and do laundry. Explain your situation first. (Check with House Cleaning in the Yellow Pages if you don't have another source. Licensing and bonding are questions you'll want to explore further before anyone new comes into your home.) *Don't expect your partner to do everything—few people can work, cook, shop, attend to a loved one confined to bed, take care of the house, and provide quality time with immediate family and the concerned extended family.*

☙ *Hire a home-care aide* if you feel you need it and can afford it. Explain your situation first. Clarify whether or not you are looking for household assistance and/or medical assistance. Many times these people can do a combination of light housekeeping, shopping, meal preparation, and laundry, as well as helping with medical and personal care and hygiene. Costs may vary, and there may be a minimum time requirement. You will probably want the same person every time for the duration of bed rest. Shop around. Personal recommendations are usually the best sources.

☙ *Home delivery services.* Find out all the delivery services that are available for your needs and desires. Explain your situation first. Suggestions:

1. Home video delivery *Note:* Videos are terrific but use discretion; some can be very stressful on nerves and cause unwanted responses, e.g. contractions, increased heart rate, etc.
2. Grocery shopping and delivery
3. Pharmacy
4. Meals (See Chapter 4: Picnics in Bed)
5. Transportation services for children
6. Dog walkers
7. Gardeners

8. Dry cleaning
9. Laundry

 Library card on hand. You've got a lot more time than ever to read. Others will be happy to pick up and deliver any book requests. Call the library ahead of time to order your books and suggest they place them in a bag for pickup.

Become a list-maker. Use paper or Post-its, pen or pencil to record items you think of that you may need immediately or in the near future. This way you won't lose track of any thoughts or ideas that need attention and execution.

Ask for help. Be prepared to answer when others ask the question, "What can I do to help?"

Important: After you have received assistance, let your helper know how much you appreciate their asking and helping. If the favor requires a purchase of any kind, let them know in advance they will be reimbursed immediately or that the payment has been prearranged.

Remember, *people like to help!* A concrete task is a favor to each individual who reaches out to you.

Be ready with a specific request.

Examples of responses:

"Thank you for asking! There are a few things around the house that I would like to have closer to me, or that I would like to check on. I have a short list, and when you come over, would you mind helping me out?"

"Thank you for asking! Would you mind picking up Bill's dry cleaning on your way. I've got money here to pay you back. It would be a huge help!"

"Thank you for asking! It would be wonderful if you came for a short visit, and while you're here would you mind watering the plants? That would be a big help today."

"Oh, I would love to have a visit, and as far as helping, it would be great! Would you mind emptying the dishwasher at some point while you're here? Every little bit makes a huge difference!"

"Oh, thank you for asking. You have such a beautiful garden. What I need more than anything today are some flowers to look at! Would you mind bringing me some from your garden? When you get here I'll tell you where you can find a vase. This is what I need more than anything else today!"

"Oh, thanks for being concerned. More than anything I just need someone to watch a video with me. Do you have the time, and would you be interested? I can have one delivered!"

Other types of errands that you'll need help with:

(*whenever possible, pay ahead with credit card or charge account*)

—Picking up groceries. Have the shopping list ready or call ahead if you have a neighborhood grocery. (Someone should be responsible for your grocery inventory list. You never want to run out of the basic necessities.) Explain your situation and ask the manager if someone can shop for the duration of your time on bed rest. Request that after you call, everything be ready by a designated time for pickup. If you don't already have a charge account, check on the possibility of opening one.

—Bringing in the mail.

—Mailing personal correspondence, bills, etc.

—Picking out gifts for special occasions. Consider asking them to have the gift wrapped with a card included.

—Shopping for art supplies and personal project supplies.

—Getting stamps at the post office (mail order option: 800-782-6724).

—Dropping off parcels at the post office.

—Picking up a child at a certain location, bringing him/

her home or providing transportation to another location whenever possible. Try to create a routine schedule involving the same driver and destination. Make sure to communicate all the details to all parties involved, especially children.

All of these errands combine visits with much-needed practical assistance.

It will help to calendar the new daily routines that emerge as a result of your bed rest. Use "The Daily Schedule" in this book to help coordinate your helpers and the various tasks.

THE ACCESSORIZED BED

Welcome to your new Command Post—your bed! It is now a central station—commonly known by bed rest veterans as "The Command Post." Your bed is also your foundation of comfort.

You may want your bed relocated, or you may consider renting a hospital bed to place somewhere else in your home. You may also consider lowering your bed closer to the floor. This is helpful if small children are involved. Diapering, climbing up, and having fun playing together is facilitated by a lower bed position. Water bed usage may require approval from your doctor.

Creating an environment that offers maximum comfort and allows for "active" living is paramount to having a positive bed rest experience. The following list of accessories is intended to help make this happen for you. The ideas will facilitate your situation by elevating your level of comfort and productivity while on bed rest:

- *Eggcrate mattress*—This is a number one priority as it is designed to reduce pressure on hips, knees, elbows, your whole body. Most medical supply stores have them, a foam mattress store carries these, and sometimes a pharmacy can order one. Refer to the Home Aid Supply Catalogs in the appendix.

- *Select comfort air mattress*—This air-supported mattress allows you to customize the firmness for each side with the touch of a button. Call 800-831-1211 for more information.
- *Bolster*—A firm back pillow that supports your back if you must lie on your side. You can either buy one or make one by taping rolled blankets (four or five usually work).
- *Lamb's-wool mattress pad*—Helps keep the body warm in winter and cool in summer. It also has a great touch to the skin.
- *Pillows*—A minimum of three. Depending on your situation, you'll want to have more available for your legs, your back and your side. Other pillows: neck support pillows (eggcrate foam), body pillows, adjustable bed wedge, leg incliner are all very therapeutic for bedridden patients. The temple pillow: a small, silk pillow for relaxing the head and forehead is available through the H2B Company in San Francisco at 415-626-REST or 800-829-6580. It can even be precooled in the freezer or refrigerator. Other relaxation pillows are available through this company. Refer to the Home Aid Supply Sources in the appendix.
- *Sheets*—Nice sheets can make a big difference! Flannel in the winter are helpful for maximizing warmth and relaxation. Bright-colored ones can help make your environment a little brighter. Smooth satin sheets allow for easy turning in bed.
- *Blankets*—Warmth is important so that your body is relaxed and focused on healing, not working to stay warm. Polar fleece material will provide warmth without the weight of a traditional wool blanket. Speak with your doctor about using an electric blanket. This may not be advisable for certain medical conditions.
- *Reading light*—You may be reading at unusual hours,

and it is important that you have plenty of light, and that you don't bother anyone if the light is on at 3 A.M.

- ◉ *Clock*—(with alarm and second hand) For scheduling medication, timing contractions, phone appointments, keeping a daily schedule.
- ◉ *Lap tray*—This tool has multiple functions: eating tray, writing surface, creative project table, computer use, reading. A six-position solid wood tray with laminate top for easy cleaning is recommended. (See Shopping Guide under Home Aid Supply Catalogs/Levenger's.)
- ◉ *Able table*—A variation of a lap tray, this adjustable, sturdy, lightweight table rests on the bed and becomes a personal workbench.
- ◉ *Overbed table with wheels*—This is a key multipurpose organizer. Ideally it is next to the bed serving as the main holding surface for items that are continually used on a daily basis. It is designed to swing over the patient's lap for ease of reach and general use. A table with an adjustable angle and height, made of wood with a stain-resistant top is highly recommended. Organization of all your personal objects reduces the burden of having everything on you and the bed. Keeping things organized and close at hand enhances personal freedom and increases energy for health and creativity! If your table is on a carpet, you may want to try a plastic carpet protector to ensure mobility of the table's wheels. (See Shopping Guide/Home Aid Supply Catalogs.)

Supplies and personal objects that belong on the overbed table:

- ❏ All medication (label the tops and sides of every vial; *always use childproof caps for the safety of your own or visiting children*)
- ❏ Telephone (recommend cordless or headset for head/neck comfort)
- ❏ Books (address book, general reading books, *The Bed Rest Survival Guide,* etc.)

- ❏ Cassette player or radio
- ❏ TV remote control
- ❏ Clock
- ❏ Pens and pencils
- ❏ Paper, Post-its, stationary
- ❏ Clipboard
- ❏ Stamps (these can be mail-ordered anytime at 800-782-6724)
- ❏ Hand cream
- ❏ Toiletries and/or makeup in cosmetic bag (mirror)
- ❏ Tissue
- ❏ Disposable hand wipes for clean hands and spills
- ❏ Walkie-talkie or other intercom device

- ◉ *Collection bin*—Always put pencils/pens, notepad, remote control, wallet, and any other small items in one place to prevent temporary and frustrating losses. Rectangular Tupperware containers or small artist's toolboxes are great for this.
- ◉ *Ice chest*—This is particularly useful if you are alone. It should contain healthful foods and drinks. (See Chapter 5: Smart and Savory Picnics.)
- ◉ *Reacher or pickerupper*—Extends your reach by picking up or suctioning objects around the bed or on the floor. Refer to appendix—Home Aid Supply Sources or call a local medical-supply store.
- ◉ *The back bar*—A therapeutic massage tool that is adjustable, compact, and light, and can be used for the neck, buttocks, hips, and back. To order or for more information, call The Outlook Design Company at 800-818-BACK. Inquire about additional product line.
- ◉ *Small fan*—Air circulation is important for simulating wind and fresh air, enhanced healing, and general productivity.
- ◉ *Bib*—Eating may be messier than usual.

BEYOND THE BED—
CREATING A PLEASANT ENVIRONMENT

- Bring the outdoors in! Ideally there is a window in your room. Maybe you've got a view! If the climate permits, keep the windows and shades wide-open. Plants and flowers help lift spirits and brighten surroundings. So do photographs of important people and special places.

- Be in good company! Attractive robes, pajamas, or loose-fitting outfits can make you look better and feel better. I wore light makeup every day of bed rest. It helped me feel better about myself. Combing or brushing your hair, shaving and putting yourself together help promote a positive attitude and handsome surroundings!

- Provide entertainment and help pass time with a television and a VCR. Get a schedule of daily or weekly TV programs and a categorized listing of videos. Don't forget the option of home video delivery. *Important: Consider the type of television and video you watch. It is recommended that you stay away from anything frightening, loud, or nerve-wracking.*

- Radio, CD, tape player provide musical and talk-show entertainment. Additionally, enjoy listening to books on tape—a restful and stimulating way to spend time.

- A cordless telephone is a must! If and when you change resting locations, bring the telephone with you. It becomes not only your connection to the outside world, but a tool for personal safety. One that has a speaker base can offer more relaxing conversations—you can let go of the receiver and just lie there and talk. Similarly, while working on the computer or other projects, you can simultaneously discuss matters while working.

- An answering machine or voice mail provides flexibility to return calls at your leisure or discretion. You may consider a message that updates your status. This way you can avoid repeating your health report if you don't feel like it.

- An intercom or walkie-talkie eliminates feeling isolated by facilitating communication throughout the house, e.g., kitchen, children's rooms, family room, or playroom.
- Reduce clutter with bookshelves. All of the many books, magazines, newspapers, and other odds and ends you collect should never pile up on the bed. Have a helper organize them on a bookshelf.
- Have a garbage container on hand. Don't let tissue, opened envelopes, etc. collect all around you. Keep your area clean and you will feel better and more productive.
- Ensure privacy with a sound screen. It's a nifty mechanical device that acts like a noice "filter." It can be used to capture unwanted background noise or to add noise if there is too much quiet in your surroundings. Refer to the Home Aid Supply Sources in the appendix/Self Care Catalog or Living Arts.
- Last but not least . . *Change* your surroundings! If you are able to change your environment by moving from your main bed to a couch, cot, or foam mattress, do it! Have an alternative bed set up in the kitchen during mealtimes, in the living room for family time or visitors, and outdoors if the weather permits. I loved talking with my husband while he cooked our dinners every evening. The cot barely fit in the room, but with a little shifting around, it worked. I also spent the majority of each day in our backyard. The sun was my best therapy for relaxation and feeling positive. There are many alternatives to lying in the same bed day after day: camp cot, inflatable raft, futon, couch, foam mattress, lounge chair, couch cushions, or plywood with pillows.

BATHROOM PRIVILEGES

For some people who are bedridden, the bedroom and bathroom are one and the same. Washing is done with wet towels and soap, or with special wipee-type cloths. The normal toilet is replaced by a bedpan, a female or male urinal (designed to reduce spillage and odor) or a bedside commode. Hair shampoos in bed may be facilitated by an inflatable or lean-back shampooer.

If you are able to walk to the bathroom, the following items offer assistance:

Safety bars—in the tub and shower and by the toilet

Transfer bench—for lowering into the tub

Bath seat—for shower or sponge bath

Contoured tall-ette toilet seat—designed for comfort and security

Bath mats—prevent slips in bath or shower

Table by the sink—if you prefer to have certain medications or other health supplements in the bathroom, e.g. vitamins, laxatives, pain relievers, or other health remedies. Toothbrush and toothpaste should also be readily available. Include a plastic cup for water.

CHAPTER THREE

Creating a Routine

Bed rest may not mean the same thing to everyone. Some people may be forced into a resting position with limited physical mobility while others may have to remain lying flat on their backs, unable to move at all. Others may be confined not only to bed, but to a hospital room, requiring very close medical attention. No matter what kind of bed rest has been prescribed for you, it is especially important to take one day at a time, remembering that each day brings you closer to reaching your goal of getting back on your feet and resuming your normal lifestyle.

During the first days of bed rest, it is easy to feel like doing absolutely nothing other than lying on the bed, drifting in and out of sleep. You may also feel unable to take care of business as usual. After some time you may begin to reorient. A daily schedule can help you feel a new sense of purpose. It will help you begin to realize that time can be well spent, even if you are stuck in bed. Soon it will become evident how much planning and daily activity there is on bed rest. A new calendar with a new daily schedule will help you feel a greater sense of confidence and stability with this new lifestyle.

THE DAILY SCHEDULE

A daily schedule can help you become an active participant in your care and your healing. Throughout the days, when you look at your schedule, ask yourself, "How am I doing?" Checking in with yourself helps you become more aware of your progress. When you have specific questions, write them down. This will remind you to share your concerns with your doctor and to ask every question you have. It helps to do everything you can to assist in your own recovery and reinforce a positive attitude. Setting goals by marking milestones on the calendar pages establishes the proper focus on healing.

Creating a schedule for yourself can help give you something to look forward to each day. This can include reading time, telephone calls, journal writing, correspondence, craft activities, personal projects, television, videos, etc.

A daily schedule helps break up your day into smaller pieces, and, before you know it, your bedridden day is very busy!

A new challenge of managing your new existence, family activities, new routines, and volunteer help will emerge as a result of being bedridden. Someday, you will look back on this time and say, how did I ever do it? Your Daily Schedule will be living proof!

Sample Routine for Your Daily Schedule:

Wake-up
Breakfast
Morning activities
Visitors/helpers
Lunch
Afternoon activities
Visitors/helpers
Dinner
Evening time

Sample Activities to Schedule:

Your professional work—time doing it, phone appoint-
  ments, etc.
Personal phone calls
Television/video/radio time
Personal projects
Personal hygiene
Doctor appointments
Daily exercise/physical therapy
Medical observations/monitoring
Special time with partner
Special time with children
Entertaining
Milestones

EXERCISE AND PHYSICAL THERAPY

Exercise and physical therapy can be a tremendous benefit to
anyone bedridden. An assessment of your situation by a professional along with an ongoing supervised program can relieve
stress. It can also manage neck, back, and joint pain, maintain
muscle strength, and reduce swelling and stiffness. It is almost
impossible to think or do anything if you cannot relax. Exercise
will make a difference.

The medical management of your bed rest is a team effort
that includes your doctors, nurses, social worker, and physical
therapist. If you are in physical pain or discomfort, physical therapy and massage will most likely be approved by your doctor.
Always consult with your doctor before doing anything that in-
volves moving your body for physical exercise.

Any program that you begin should be a personalized one.
Once you begin, it is important that you be aware of the impact of
physical movement on your body. If at any time the exercises make
you feel uncomfortable (in the case of pregnancy you feel increased
contractions or in the case of a back injury you feel increased pain),

Daily Schedule

Monday	9:00 Check-in phone call with Dr. Hansen 10:00 Call the Office, check e-mail 12:00 Lunch with Patty—Chinese	3:30 Order Video delivery 4:00 Massage with Trisha 7:00 Dick home—dinner and video
Tuesday	8:00 Shower! (wash hair) 9:00 Check voice mail and e-mail 11:30 Physical Therapy appt. *ask her to bring lunch before she leaves 12:30 Letters to friends with new medical update.	3:00 Visit from Dee and Karin— they're bringing dinner! 4:00 Finish library book and put in pile/must return tomorrow! 7:00 Dick home—he just has to warm up dinner.
Wednesday	8:00 Start Photo Album Project 10:00 Physical therapy appt. 11:30 Lynne arrives with mail, groceries and lunch. 1:00 Telephone Conference Call with Department Heads	3:30 Relax with video—do exercises while viewing 5:30 Read magazines, newspaper, etc. 7:00 Dinner—Dick heats leftovers
Thursday	8:00 Photo Project 9:30 Check-in phone call with Dr. Hansen 11:30 Physical therapy appt.—Give her outgoing letters to mail.	12:30 Dick home for lunch 5:00 Call Dick with list of groceries

Daily Schedule

Friday

8:00 Shower!
9:30 Check Voice Mail and e-mail
11:00 Exercises
11:45 Cleaning lady:
   -new bed sheets
   -take letters to mail

12:30 Relax with nature video
2:30 Photo Albums—FINISH!
5:00 Call Sushi and order take out
6:00 Dick home

Saturday

10:00 Massage from Trisha
12:00 Visit from David and Elizabeth
1:00 Dick to knitting store to pick
   up supplies

6:30 Emmy over for dinner/pizza
   and salad

Sunday

Cot outside for sunny
morning
Dick—gardening. Knitting and
NY Times for me.

stop doing the exercises until you check with your doctor. If you are on medication that is known to increase your heart rate and cause shortness of breath, you need to be especially aware that your heart rate does not exceed 120 beats per minute at any time.

Limited exercise has tremendous benefits for anyone confined to bed rest. Even exercise that may seem trivial at first can save you from atrophy that will occur more quickly than you might realize. Light exercise will maintain muscle tone and circulation during the time you are required to be still and in bed. (Stay attuned to your body. Stay in close communication with your physician and physical therapist.) Too much exercise or the wrong kind of exercise can cause unnecessary difficulties and present barriers to wellness. A reminder: check with your insurance carrier about coverage for physical therapy, massage, exercise equipment, etc. You may be delighted to learn that much of your care is paid for by your carrier. You may also discover that you are heading into a managed program that, if not covered by insurance, may be financially prohibitive.

For anyone on bed rest, it is helpful to do an exercise program at a regular time each day (ten to twenty minutes in the morning and the same in the afternoon). Adding music while exercising can help make each session enjoyable and different.

If you are pregnant and on bed rest, it is normally recommended that you *not* do any exercises that use muscles in the abdominal region. Doctors advise against doing any squats or holding your breath. Even mild exercise can cause contractions.

Suggestions for simple exercises (doctor's approval first):

Breathing (not for pregnant patients)
Sitting or lying down, depending on your prescribed position, begin with ten deep inhalations/exhalations held to ten seconds each. The breathing exercises help strengthen the chest muscles.

Isometrics
Isometric exercises can be done with any muscle group

of the body. Depending on where your injury is, exclude the muscles in that sensitive area. In the case of pregnancy, don't use your abdominal muscles. Tighten and loosen each muscle group: face, neck, back, shoulders, arms, hands, thighs, calves, and feet. You may try to press your hands and feet against the headboard, footboard, or wall. Isometrics maintain circulation and muscle tone.

After the isometrics, loosen up each set of joints by rotating: neck, shoulders, arms, hands, feet.

Stretching

Remaining in your prescribed bed rest position for all exercises:

Neck stretches—Tilt your head to the left as far as possible without strain, keeping shoulders level and relaxed; then to the right side. Repeat ten times with each side.

Neck rotation—Keeping your shoulders level and relaxed, place your left hand on your left cheek, pushing gently with your hand while resisting slightly with your cheek. Turn your head as far to the right as you can, without strain. Then reverse and use your right hand and your right cheek. Repeat ten times on each side.

Shoulder stretch—Raise your left shoulder toward your left ear as far as possible without tilting your head, then relax your shoulder completely and drop. Switch to right side. Repeat two sets of ten with each side.

Shoulder roll—Roll both shoulders up and forward as high and as far forward as possible, then reverse. Do six times each way.

Chest and Arms

Arm press—Lift your arms in front of you at right angles to your chest at nipple height. Bending your arms, press your palms together firmly. Push together and relax. Do two sets of ten.

Arm lift—Extend your arms fully out in front of you at about shoulder level, using either very light weights or canned goods of the same weight. With your arms still extended, lift your arms up slowly above your chest and head, then back down toward the bed slowly. Repeat one to two sets of ten.

Biceps press—Holding the weights in your hands, and your arms extended fully in front of you at shoulder level, bend your arms at the elbows, bringing your hands to the shoulder, working the biceps. Repeat at least two sets of ten.

Wrist press—Extending your arms forward, palms up, hold weights in your hands, supporting the extended arms on pillows. Bend the arm at the wrist, bringing the hand toward the forearm as far as possible, holding the weights in the hand. Do one to two sets of ten, focusing on the forearms.

Hand grip—Use a hand grip, available at sporting good stores, an Eggcerciser (in HomeAid Catalogs), or use a hard rubber ball, tennis ball, or racquet ball. Squeeze as tightly as possible. You will build up your forearms.

Wrist rotation—Raise each arm and do wrist circles in each direction several times.

Legs

Leg lift—Turn on your left side with your right leg stacked on top of your left leg, supporting your body with your right arm. Lift your right leg at a forty-five-degree angle with the foot flexed, pointing your toe slightly downward. Do two sets of ten. Repeat on the right side, lifting left leg.

Ankle circles—On your side, lift your leg in the air and do ankle circles, flexing your foot as you come up and pointing your foot as you circle down. This is good for calf muscles. Repeat on the opposite side.

Hamstring and back combo stretch—Lying on your back, pull you left leg toward your chest. Keep the other leg as straight as possible, without straining. Do this to both sides. This will help slowly to loosen up the hamstrings and back muscles.

Whole leg stretch—On your back, bend your left knee, bringing your thigh to your abdomen, and then extend your left leg, flexing your foot. Keep the other leg as straight as possible. Hold your flex ten seconds or longer if you are comfortable and not straining. Repeat several times. Repeat with your right leg.

Kegel Exercises
(especially important during pregnancy bed rest)

Kegel exercises are designed to strengthen the muscles surrounding the bladder and the vagina, both of which are stretched during the normal course of pregnancy. These exercises are useful both before and after birth.

Whether you are lying flat, sitting or standing (post bed-rest), tighten the muscles around the vagina, and hold them tightly for three to five seconds. Release. Repeat between twenty and a hundred times per day. (To be sure that you are doing the exercises properly, imagine you are trying to stop the stream of urine when urinating.)

After you have completed your exercises it is very important to do three things: relax, breathe deeply, and drink a large glass of water, juice, or whatever you desire to quench your thirst.

GETTING THROUGH THE NIGHT

Insomnia, a common problem in pregnancy and for people without physical activity, can be intensified if you are on bed rest. Tension, anxiety, indigestion, or other discomforts can make it hard to fall asleep. If you are on medication around the clock, you may be forced to wake up several times during the night. If you are in a different room than usual, or in a different bed, such as a rented hospital bed, sleeping soundly may require a major adjustment. Try some easy home remedies to help yourself relax before bedtime.

- Warm milk
- A light snack
- A warm shower (if allowed)
- A heating pad or hot water bottle in bed with you
- A gentle massage

- ⑥ Relaxing music
- ⑥ Earplugs

Avoid the following:

- ⑥ Stimulants after twilight, e.g. coffee, tea, sodas, chocolate, smoking.
- ⑥ Unnecessary medications that interfere with sleep. Discuss with your doctor if you suspect your medication is causing sleeplessness.
- ⑥ Difficult phone conversations or discussions with family or friends.
- ⑥ Working yourself into a frenzy fearing that you won't fall asleep.

Practice Relaxation Techniques

The harder you try to sleep, the harder it is to fall asleep, especially when you've been relatively still all day. Relaxing your mind and body is the best way to teach yourself how to fall asleep. Here are some techniques that experts have found particularly successful:

- ⑥ Slow down your breathing and imagine the air moving slowly in and out of your body while you breathe from your diaphragm.
- ⑥ Concentrate on relaxing your body one part at a time. Start with your toes, your feet, your ankles—and work your way up. Go slowly.
- ⑥ Program yourself to turn off unpleasant thoughts as they creep into your mind. To do that, think about enjoyable experiences that you've had. Reminisce about good times, fantasize, or play some mental games. Try counting sheep or counting backwards from one thousand by sevens.

CHAPTER FOUR

Bedside Entertainment and Personal Projects

Your room should be accessible to your family and friends but should remain the place where your comfort and stillness have the utmost priority. It should not be a place that becomes too loud or invites so much activity that you become hyper or anxiety-ridden. Family and friends must understand and respect the limitations of bed rest before you invite them to jump in and have a great time.

Along these same lines, the room should be childproof so that everyone can maximize the time together and not worry about potential disasters.

Here are ideas for playing games independently or with others of any age. Games that are played on the bed should be lightweight, should not require physical effort, or contain spillable liquids. Have fun!

BED GAMES

Checkers
Backgammon

Chess
Chinese checkers
Mancala
Cards
Jigsaw puzzles
Crossword puzzles
Coloring books
Modeling clay
Model building
Reading joke books (laughter is one of the best medicines available!)
Reading riddle books
Viewing videos or special television shows
Fun activities with children
Group reading (plays, storytelling, short stories, novels, newspaper)
Hugs and tickling (very small children love the "Tickle Monster")
Board games (Scrabble, Monopoly, Clue, Candy Land, etc.)
Sing-along music tapes
Read-along book tapes
Cat's cradle and other string games
Finger songs, e.g. "Itsy-Bitsy Spider," "London Bridge"
Finger puppets
Hand shadows
Puppet dolls and puppet shows

A great resource is a new book (1996), *Fun Time, Family Time* (Avon Books) by Susan Perry.

PERSONAL PROJECTS

Keeping busy is good therapy. And now you've got more time than ever before to rediscover old hobbies and explore new ones.

Initially, the adjustment to this radically different lifestyle is overwhelming. The first days of bed rest are usually spent reading, talking on the phone, and resting. However, after a while, you will probably feel ready to refocus your attention on other things.

Here are some suggestions of how to spend time quietly while being creative and productive. These ideas will offer a whole range of opportunities—many of which you might not have otherwise thought about. While writing this chapter, I had a strange yearning for my bed rest days. I hope my suggestions energize your journey in making the most of your time in bed. Try not to deny yourself a certain type of activity if it sounds like it would be more appropriate for the opposite gender. I can't tell you how many guys on my college ski team knitted while we traveled from race to race. Throughout my swim-team years, many of the male swimmers beaded flower chain necklaces and wove macramé belts. The creative outlet gave them something very special.

Please don't expect to do everything on the following lists. Be sensitive to the importance of balancing stimulation and stillness. Enjoy!

Reading

- Every book by an author.
- Specific literary categories, e.g. romance, mysteries, poetry, science fiction.
- Nonfiction categories: biographies, dogs, psychology, self-help, health, business, child care, history, pop culture, career development.
- Your child's schoolbooks.
- Every book on your bookshelf.
- Daily and weekly newspapers—subscribe to international newspapers, e.g. *New York Times,* the *International Herald Tribune,* etc. (See list in Shopper's Guide, at the end of this chapter.)
- Medical books on your physical condition.

- Take a correspondence course and work toward a new degree.
- Travel books. Map books, atlases.
- Cookbooks.
- Cartoon books, joke books, riddle books.
- Baby name books (particularly if you're on pregnancy bed rest).
- Software documentation and general computer information literature.
- Local community history documents.
- All your old letters.
- Go through all of your saved magazines and clip articles, recipes, designs, etc. for files.

Recorded Books

Recorded Books, Inc. provides unabridged single-voice performances on book-packaged cassettes, featuring the very best books in- and out-of-print, available for both rental and purchase, by mail. For more information and a free catalog, call 1-800-638-1304.

Writing

- Journal writing is a terrific way to express thoughts and feelings about what's going on in your life. My bed rest journal contains recordings of every day of my three-month experience. It helped me through the many hours of being alone. Whenever I had difficult moments, I turned to my bed rest journal. When I had positive news from a doctor's appointment I wrote in my journal. Processing my feelings through writing helped me get through each day. I encourage you to keep a journal. It will be a treasure to read months and years later.

- Postcards, letters, or notes to your partner, children, new baby, relatives, friends, and work associates is a great way to communicate whatever you would like to share with these important people in your life. Words of appreciation and expressions of love make you and others feel good. Medical updates will be a constant source of interest to everyone in your life. Whenever I wrote to anyone, I used a piece of carbon paper so that I could keep a copy to include in my bed rest journal.
- Authoring your own short stories, screenplays, comics, poems, novels.
- Songwriting with musical accompaniment.
- Letters to the editors in newspapers and magazines.
- Make or revise your will. If you are on pregnancy bed rest, take the new baby(s) into account.
- Write to someone you don't know, e.g. people in other

Dear Julie,
Thanks so much for your package! The books are very appreciated! I spend most of my late afternoons reading and relaxing. So far, bedrest has been a time to catch up on the many projects that have been neglected for years. It's quite amazing how much time there is in the day when you're just having to stay put. Would you ever have imagined—me on bedrest?!!!

Please stay in close touch—
Love, Barb

JULIE CHILDS
409 Main Street
Amherst, FL
40203

JOURNAL

February 22, 1987

Two weeks of bedrest has passed and I am surviving. I could never have imagined myself being able to endure this for more than a day but it's not that terrible. The key for me is to stay busy and I'm somehow able to find many things to occupy my time. I find I enjoy organizing my day and Dick's day with lists of things to do, things that the house needs or that I need. We got the laptop figured out so I can access e-mail any time. That whole process, turning the computer on and reading and responding to e-mails eats up a lot of time. The work thing makes me very tired. I'm not sure how long I can maintain my focus. It feels more exhausting to me under these conditions.

Thank god I can take a shower twice a week. The hot water feels so good on my body. Five minutes isn't nearly long enough but it boosts my spirits so I shouldn't complain. I'm realizing that bed rest probably won't kill me. It's going to be tough, but there's no choice. I feel the best when someone comes to visit me. I wonder how long this will last. I do like my quiet time, too. When visitors leave, I feel a dip in my mood when I'm left alone. I try not to dwell on this and get quickly absorbed in a video, phone calls, knitting or reading. I'm trying to hard to keep my chin up. This is not time to feel sorry for myself. I would sink too low if I dwelled on it. I've got to be strong.

February 23, 1989

It was a sunny day today. The blossoms are so beautiful outside my window. I wish I could dance around outside. No way this Spring. I'm a little down today. I literally have to force myself to accept being bedridden and focus on the physical therapy exercises, reading good books, preparing my snacks from the "snackbar" on my bed and knowing I have lots of support. I wish I didn't get so hungry—I don't want to blow up while being so inactive. I must tell Dick no fattening foods on my cooler and no treats—even though he provides them as a gesture of affection. I wouldn't mind some new eating habits and I think I'm on my way. I've never enjoyed carrot sticks and rice cakes so much!

JOURNAL

February 24, 1989

It's Friday and the weekend is upon us. I know I won't be going anywhere but right here but at least Dick will be home and maybe some other people will come visit. Today I am anticipating Dick going out without me tonight. It's Blair's birthday party and he should go. I want to be a good sport about it. I am trying to be strong and accept this predicament.

February 25, 1989

I had my first big cry last night. I lost control when Dick came home from the party. I was trying to be strong but I felt so frustrated! I wanted to scream but I cried and cried and cried. Once I did this, I felt fine again. I realize that it's o.k.—even healthy—to let it all out once in a while. It's part of finding the strength to endure this kind of continuous stillness.

countries (pen pal), a political figure (support a cause), charity organizations, etc.

 Volunteer to address envelopes for local organizations.

 Calligraphy—learn from a how-to-book.

 Become ambidextrous—If you are right-handed, teach yourself how to write with your left hand, or the other way around.

Crafts

Needlework:

This kind of craftwork is great for keeping hands active and minds and eyes focused on something colorful and rewarding. There's nothing like a finished product—either enjoying it yourself (a crocheted afghan or hand-knit sweater) or giving it away as a gift (beaded bracelets and necklaces, knitted vests, macramé wall hangings, etc.). Pace yourself and avoid hand, arm, or wrist strain. Muscular strain can lead to carpal tunnel syndrome. There is no need to invite any more physical limitations.

 Knitting: whether knitting colorful squares for a baby blanket, coordinated vests for the entire family, a complicated Norwegian ski sweater, socks, hats, or new Christmas stockings, this craft is very rewarding.

 Sewing: choosing something that can lie out in front of you, that isn't too complicated, and allows for hand sewing (small portable sewing machines may work depending on your position), sewing is the answer to occupying well-utilized time. Dolls, doll clothing, shorts, shirts, ties, quilts, scarves, etc., are within a reasonable size range.

 Needlepoint: pillows, a picture for the baby's room, bookmarks, eyeglass case, or a sign that says "Sleeping" to hang over the doorknob of your own bedroom. This is a very pleasant activity.

 Stitchery: kits are available at most craft centers. A hoop

to brace the material is highly recommended to reduce strain on arms and hands.

- Embroidery: a fine needle and colorful thread allow you to transform napkins, tablecloths, shirts, jeans into custom artistry.
- Crocheting: with a skein of yarn and one small hook, you'll be amazed how quickly you can create something useful. Crocheted afghans, hats, and vests are very popular. This is probably the easiest needlework and least strain on your arms and hands.
- Rug Hooking: latch-hook rugs are easy and lightweight. You can hook by hand or with a special hook. This is something you can do with the help of others.
- Beadwork: the possibilities are endless with beads. To get started, you can use dental floss and a sewing needle. Elastic string is ideal for making necklaces, bracelets, anklets, earrings, hairpieces, etc. Buttons, pieces of worn glass, letter cubes, shells, raw pasta, large and small beads can be beaded. Safety-pin bracelets are exquisite pieces of jewelry. Important advice: keep all beads in containers so that you do not end up sharing your bed with them.

Other Crafts:

- Model-making: from cars to horses, the possibilities are endless. Make sure your room is well ventilated if you are using glues or epoxies.
- Candle-making: small or large candles can be beautifully adorned with strips, cut-out shapes and textured clumps of colorful wax. Natural or colored beeswax candles are easy to make. Candles are nice as gifts or for home entertaining and decoration.
- Macramé: this activity is also great arm and hand exercise. You can make belts, dog or cat collars, planters, jewelry, wall hangings, and more.
- Woodworking with small pieces of wood is advisable, even for bedresters who have experience with tools and carving wood. I read about a hospitalized pregnancy case

where the woman made a baby step stool, sanding precut pieces and painting and varnishing it, all while lying in bed. Someone else who was bedridden made beautiful woodcuts in bed. The carving, inking, and printing was all done from a reclining position. Suggestion: use sharp utensils with great care and only if you have a lot of previous experience; use a plastic bag under and over your body to prevent wood chips from getting inside your clothing or bed. If you are pregnant, consult with your doctor before using glue, varnish, or other materials that might have toxic fumes.

- Jewelry: there are kits available for silver and gold jewelry-making. They contain necklace latches, earring bases and backs, glue, thread for beading, and all kinds of beads. This is the best way to get started while you are on bed rest unless you are experienced and already have supplies. Great for keeping yourself well adorned and for handmade gifts.

Some excellent resources for crafts:
1. Curiosity Kits—makers of premade craft packages.
Curiosity Kits, P.O. Box 811, Cockeysville, MD 21030
Phone: 800-584-KITS E-mail: Ckitsinc@aol.com
2. Klutz Press @ 415-424-0739 or www.klutz.com

BECOMING AN ARTIST

When else would you ever have this much privacy or time to express yourself artistically? Have you ever experimented with art, enjoyed it, had a good laugh or felt very satisfied and then never followed through to explore your talent? Have you ever had the urge to drop everything for a while and tap into your creative nature? Here is your chance.

- Drawing: What could be simpler? You will need plain paper or sketch pad, pencils, and an eraser. Add to the possibilities with colored pencils, crayons, watercolors, charcoal, paints, and small canvases. Bookstores, art stores, and libraries are good sources for beginning or technical drawing guides. Or, try tracing family photos or magazine pictures. Get an adult paint or pencil by number kit. Another possibility is fabric painting. You can draw, write, color-in anything. Fabric painting is a simple, easy-to-use way to hand-decorate household items. You can put your personal touch on sweatshirts, T-shirts, shoes (sneakers are best), baby bibs, dolls, lunch boxes, etc. I use fabric paints and acrylics to decorate flowerpots. Suggestion for wet work: use a plastic garbage bag on the lap tray and either wear a plastic smock or put another garbage bag under your body to protect the bed.

◉ Clay: Have someone deliver a good-size hunk of clay to your bedside. Always keep it in plastic to preserve the necessary moisture for kneading and sculpting. Whenever you feel like sculpting something, take it out and mold away. Jewelry and pottery can be made with Fimo dough and other ceramic clays. There are many good books available on creativity with clay. Some books even come with colorful clay samples. Get the specifics on how to maintain the clay so you don't get discouraged or waste time and money by using it incorrectly. Use a plastic garbage bag on the lap tray and either wear a plastic smock or put another garbage bag under your body to protect the bed. Be forewarned, many clays have a fairly strong odor. Hopefully this won't be a problem for you.

◉ Photography: If this is something you've always wanted to do, invest your time in reading everything there is to know about the art and science of photography. When you are off bed rest, you will be an expert, prepared and ready to set up a darkroom and begin your photographic journey. While in bed, you can experiment with camera and film, trying techniques and analyzing the effects by having the film processed elsewhere. You may also enjoy teaching yourself the art of color-tinting old black-and-white photos. To begin, ask someone to bring you black-and-white photocopies of a favorite photograph to practice and test your sense of color. When you are ready, collect actual photos and begin doing the real thing. You may find you have a side business in the making, perhaps while you are still bedridden.

 Paper art: Teach yourself origami, the art of paper-folding. There are excellent books on the market, some of which include special paper for getting started. Paper chains, paper airplanes, paper dolls, paper houses, paper snowflakes, paper cutouts of all kinds are a fun way to spend time. You don't have to have little ones around to enjoy this lost art. Make your own note cards, postcards, birthday cards. Suggestion—Use glue sticks rather than glue in a bottle. *Do not* use super glues unless your room is well ventilated.

 Photo albums and scrapbooks: These are creative ventures that require few tools and can occupy large blocks of time. Scrapbooks can be used for anything: baby books, recipes, photo journals, personal correspondence. If your photos are like most people's photos, they are overabundant, disorganized, and stashed away in envelopes with the intention that someday they will be put into photo albums. Here's your chance finally to do it!

The trick to making headway:

1. Get organized by collecting all the photos.
2. Order the photos by year, month, and day. Tip: Use old calendars to jog your memory.
3. Have someone buy photo albums. Be specific as to the size, format, and number of albums. Hint: Buy inexpensive photo albums with many pages. If you care about how they look on your bookshelf or on a coffee table, cover them with nice fabric or fancy paper. This is what I do, and now I have volumes of very attractive photo albums.
4. Mount the photos. If there are no plastic pockets for

easy insertion, use glue sticks or the traditional mounting triangles and apply to the page wherever you think the photo looks best.

5. For labeling and chronicling events and time periods, correction tape works as little comment strips, or cut your own narrow pieces of paper. The strips can then be glued onto the pages in any location.

6. When you have extra photos from one scene and are unwilling to discard any one of them (this is always my dilemma), cut out the essential parts of the photo (around a person's head and body or around two people, the dog and the beautiful side garden. Through a collage effect, this technique produces movement on the page. It also saves space and makes for fun viewing.

◉ Graphics and illustration software is the high-tech approach to artistry. If you are using a laptop for work, you can add artistic programs for a creative outlet. Broderbund Software, Adobe, and Microsoft have superb software for drawing, painting, graphics, card-making, etc.

RESEARCH FAMILY TREE

What a great opportunity to delve into researching your family tree! Call or write to extended family members, use the Internet, and pursue alternative resources through the local library.

SOUNDS OF MUSIC

◉ Learn to play a musical instrument. It is never too late to learn how to play or read notes. If you already play an instrument and it's light enough and can be held properly while you are bedridden, do it! If you normally play the cello and there's no way to continue while on bed rest, try a ukulele or a completely different instrument. Try an electronic keyboard. It is narrow enough to fit next to you if you are on your side, or it can be placed on a lap tray. Keyboards are sold everywhere these days, including mass-merchandise stores like Costco and Kmart. For beginners, basic music theory books and self-teaching books are available in local music stores. Words of caution: Playing an instrument takes a lot of energy, especially from a reclining position. Observe your breathing and heart rate, as you do not want to increase either to an undesired point.

- Listen to music on tape, compact disc, radio, or television. Headphones may enhance activity. If you normally listen to one type of music, such as jazz or rock, try listening to classical, country, or opera. You may discover a whole new world of musical enjoyment.

- Listen to and watch famous symphonies, ballet, or opera performances on video or television. This is a great way to lift one's spirits while being passive and restful.

- Make a mix on a cassette for someone or for yourself using a CD player and cassette or dual cassette player/recorder.

PERSONAL FINANCES

This may be the time to further your knowledge or level of involvement with your personal finances. It may be that you are just a beginner. Here's the chance to begin to organize your finances, review your budget plan, and consider investment opportunities. The business section of newspapers, financial publications (*Wall Street Journal, Money Magazine,* etc.), books, accountants, and banks offer a bounty of material for your use. Home banking, on line bill paying and account information can be fulfilled by the Internet. Ask your bank if they have this capability and to provide you with the necessary information, e.g. web site addresses. For bill paying, I suggest www.checkfree.

com. This is a great time to invite your accountant or financial advisor to visit you at home.

FILING

*O*rganize your personal files: automobile maintenance, banking, credit cards, insurance policies, newspaper articles of interest, legal material, résumé, personal correspondence, creative writing, decorating ideas, home projects, warranties, etc.

LAPTOP PROJECTS

*O*nce you're hooked up to a computer, your opportunities are virtually limitless (a more detailed Computer Guide can be found later in this chapter). With the wide range of available software packages, you can explore projects ranging from graphic design and illustration, to tax preparation or newsletter production.

On the Internet, you can download everything you've ever wanted to know about any subject: sports or travel, art history or politics—it's *all* there. You can join chat sessions with your local news reporters or you can "talk" to physicians about your medical problem!

The best way to get acquainted with what's available on the Internet is to start with a search service such as Yahoo (www.yahoo.com). Enter any subject of interest into the search text box and it will return a list of sites that reference that interest. Exploring the multitude of topics available on line can keep you busy for as long as you are interested.

The time spent on the Internet costs money, so you will want to find a provider that offers a monthly plan that suits your budget. **Remember to disconnect after each use; otherwise, you will be charged for the time.** Don't forget to visit my web site at www.bedrest.com.

There is an ocean of software on almost any subject matter (available by mail order). Tutorial books, tapes, and videos for enhancing your knowledge are available at libraries, bookstores, and computer outlets.

PERSONAL TIME

Rarely in life do we have idle time. You may find many moments of bed rest that are. Why not take these moments as the chance to do the personal things you never have time for. Here are some ideas:

- Trim your own hair (prior experience advised), or have a professional visit for a cut and style
- Give yourself a facial, or have a professional visit to give you one
- Give yourself a manicure, or have a professional or friend visit to do your hands and feet
- Experiment with makeup
- Meditate
- Sing or chant
- Record your voice, listen and explore your tones and inflections
- Self-massage
- Study acupressure and try it on yourself (see reference charts in Appendix F)
- Talk to yourself in a mirror and explore how others see you

COMPUTER GUIDE

Although computers can be rather costly if you don't already have one, they're a great educational and personal investment as well as allowing the most ideal use of time for someone who is bedridden. Computers and the Internet provide a myriad of opportunities. They are educational, interactive, creative, and offer something for everyone. Additionally, you can connect with millions of other people who also spend their time on the computer—some of whom may be fellow bedresters!

While many other resources go into more detail, here are some basics for how to get started.

Computer:

On bed rest, if you don't already have a laptop, try to get one. They are so much more manageable for your bed environment than trying to use a desktop computer. A laptop fits well on an able table or lap tray. Laptops can be rented or borrowed. If someone can help you, they can also be purchased at a mass-merchandising store like CompUSA, Fry's, or Costco for less than $2,000. Another option is to order your equipment through one of the reputable mail-order companies.* You may get better service, better pricing, and better technical support going this route. Traditionally, mail-order companies bundle software, which generally includes everything that you'd immediately need to get started. Finally, you might look into refurbished or used laptops for a good deal. Technology is advancing so rapidly that "old" models of computers may be only one year old and just fine for your purposes. Again, if someone is available to do the pickup, you can find listings of refurbished or used computers in your local newspaper, free computer magazines, or mail-order catalogs. Depending on what you decide, you will spend somewhere between one and four thousand dollars.

Virtually every laptop made runs one of two operating systems: Windows or Macintosh. The Macintosh has been renowned for its easy-to-use interface. The latest version of Windows, Windows 95, is equally easy and intuitive. More than 90 percent of personal computers now use Windows and, as a result, there is more software available for this operating system. A 486 or better processor is recommended for a Windows compatible laptop and a 64040 or Power PC processor is recommended for a Macintosh laptop. Whether Windows or Macintosh, the following is recommended: 32 megabytes of RAM, at least a gigabyte of hard disk space and a color screen (800×600 display). (Seeing beautiful graphics is half the fun these days; however, color adds considerably to the cost of a laptop computer).

Modem:

Modems are necessary if you want to connect to the Internet (includes the use of e-mail) or to other people's computers. Modems translate what is in your computer and send it over your normal telephone line. The modem at the other end retranslates the phone signal back into information that goes on the other person's computer. The higher the speed of the modem, the faster data will come into your computer (and thus the faster it will draw on your monitor). Therefore, the recommendation is to get at least a 33.6k modem. Modems can either be internal (boards put inside the computer) or external (boxes that sit outside and are linked to the back of the computer). The easiest route is to get a computer that already has a modem built into it.

CD-ROM:

A CD ROM is a peripheral device that allows you to take advantage of the best entertainment and educational software available. The graphics in these programs require a huge amount of storage space, which can only be held by CD-ROM.

Printer:

Once you have a computer, chances are you'll want a printer. You have two choices: a laser printer or inkjet printer. A laser printer is faster and generally the print is of higher quality than that of the inkjet printer. The major advantage of the inkjet is that you have the option of getting color for much less expense than a color laser printer.

Communication software:

The modem needs a program to tell it how to translate all this data and how to talk to other computers and the Internet. Internet communication software will perform this function. But first you need to find a company to give you the link to the Internet and the software you need to connect to the Internet.

Software:

You cannot do anything with your computer unless you have software to run the various programs you're interested in. There is a good chance that whatever system you obtain will include software. Nowadays, you don't have to worry about getting yourself started from ground zero. It's all very user-friendly. If you're unaware of all the different types of software available, call one of the mail-order companies and request a catalog. You'll marvel at the thousands of options. Enjoy!

Internet account:

There are many ways to get an individual account to link to the Internet. The company that has the host computer that you will link to is called an internet service provider. Typically your service provider will give you the communication software you need with your account. For individual accounts, choose what is called a SLIP (Serial Line Interface Protocol), or PPP (Point to Point Protocol) account.

You may choose either a commercial online service or a private service provider. The advantages of the larger providers is their services include technical support, easy-to-use interfaces, and special offerings unique to their service. Private service providers offer the links to the Internet only. They do not add a lot of fancy services. They focus more on providing cost-effective connections rather than building their own proprietary networks and information sources. The advantage of these services is their typical flat-fee-per-month cost rather than the per-hour connect fees of the commercial services. There's a lot of competition in this area so shop around.

When you make it on-line, visit our web site: www.bedrest. com. There is a chat capability waiting to be utilized. Your story may be of great interest to someone else on bed rest with a similar medical problem or reaction to bed rest. On-line connectivity can break the barrier of geographic distances.

Recommended mail order companies:
(Most mail order offers both sides: PC and Macintosh)

1. MicroWarehouse (PC) 1-800-367-7080
   MacWarehouse (Mac) 1-800-255-6227
2. PC and Mac Connection 1-800-800-1111
3. Computer Discount Warehouse (CDW) 1-800-557-4239
4. Multiple Zones International (''Mac or PC Zone'') 1-800-248-0800
5. Tiger Software Mac Products 1-800-666-2562
   PC Products 1-800-888-4437
6. Educational Resources 1-800-624-2926
7. Educational Software Institute 1-800-955-5570
8. Learning Services 1-800-877-9378

SHOPPER'S GUIDE

Shopping by telephone and mail order:

For *serious* shoppers, the AT&T Toll Free 800 Directory is an efficient way to obtain categorized names of companies, addresses, and 800 numbers for fulfilling many of your shopping needs. These directories list companies alphabetically **by business category.** Call 800-222-0400 to order:

- *The Consumer Shopper's Guide* ($14.95)—lists over 60,000 retailers and home-convenience companies.
- *The Business Edition* ($19.95)—lists over 120,000 wholesalers and manufacturers.
- Both editions can be purchased for $29.95.
- The CD-ROM edition is available for $19.95.

For clothing and household basics:

- L.L. Bean 1-800-514-2326 (clothes, lightweight cots, ''camping'' items)
- Land's End 1-800-356-4444 (clothes)
- Williams Sonoma 1-800-541-2233 (kitchen)
- Chambers 1-800-334-9790 (robes, sheets, etc.)

- The Company Store 1-800-285-3696 (pillows, mattresses, sheets, towels)
- Eddie Bauer Home 1-800-426-8020 (clothes and household accessories)
- HomeOffice 1-800-869-6000 (office supplies)
- Sky Mall 1-800-SKY-MALL (appliances, gadgets/toys, clothes)

For children and babies—clothing (including maternity), books, toys, safety and educational supplies, baby basics:

- Hearth Song 1-800-325-2502 (books, toys, creative projects)
- After the Stork 1-800-441-4775 (clothes, baby accessories)
- Biobottoms 1-800-766-1254 (clothes, baby accessories)
- Hannah Anderson 1-800-222-0544 (clothes, baby accessories)
- Playclothes 1-800-654-6839 (clothes, costumes)
- ChildCraft 1-800-631-5657 (clothes, costumes)
- Sensational Beginnings 1-800-444-2147 (baby accessories, toys, clothes)
- One Step Ahead 1-800-274-8440 (baby accessories, toys, clothes)
- Hand in Hand 1-800-872-9745 (toys, educational tools, safety accessories)
- The Natural Baby Catalog 1-609-771-9342 (clothes and accessories)

For health care and home aid supply catalogs:

- Mountainville House Calls 1-800-460-7282 (household/health-care accessories)
- BackSaver 1-800-251-2225 (furniture and accessories)
- Living Arts 1-800-254-8464 (clothes, health accessories)
- Self Care 1-800-345-3371 (household and health-care remedies)
- Levenger 1-800-544-0880 (furniture, able table, overbed tables, etc.)
- Hold Everything 1-800-421-2264 (household organizers)

- ⊚ Anderson Bedroom Organizer 1-800-782-4825 (household organizers)
- ⊚ Hands-On Health Care Catalog 1-800-442-2232 (healthcare accessories)
- ⊚ Frontgate 1-800-626-6488 (general household furniture/accessories)

For magazine subscriptions:
- ⊚ *Audubon* 1-800-274-4201
- ⊚ *Better Homes & Garden* 1-800-374-4244
- ⊚ *Black Enterprise* 1-800-727-7777
- ⊚ *Business Week* 1-800-635-1200
- ⊚ *Computer Life* 1-800-926-1578
- ⊚ *Ebony* 1-312-322-9200
- ⊚ *The Economist* 1-800-456-6086
- ⊚ *Elle* 1-800-876-8775
- ⊚ *Entertainment Weekly* 1-800-541-1000
- ⊚ *Family Life* 1-303-604-1464
- ⊚ *Financial Times* 1-800-628-8088
- ⊚ *Forbes* 1-800-888-9896
- ⊚ *Fortune* 1-800-541-1000
- ⊚ *Gourmet* 1-800-888-8728
- ⊚ *Harper's* 1-800-444-4653
- ⊚ *Home* 1-303-604-1464
- ⊚ *In Style* 1-800-274-6200
- ⊚ *Inc.* 1-800-234-0999
- ⊚ *International Herald Tribune* 1-800-882-2884
- ⊚ *Internet World* 1-800-573-3062
- ⊚ *Investor's Business Daily* 1-800-831-2525
- ⊚ *Ladies' Home Journal* 1-800-374-4545
- ⊚ *Mac Home Journal* 1-800-800-6542
- ⊚ *Money Magazine* 1-800-541-1000
- ⊚ *National Geographic* 1-800-NGS-LINE
- ⊚ *Nation's Business* 1-800-873-4769
- ⊚ *New Republic* 1-800-827-1289
- ⊚ *New Yorker* 1-800-825-2510
- ⊚ *New York Times* 1-800-631-2500

- *Newsweek* 1-800-631-1040
- *The Nikon Keizai Shimbun* 1-800-322-1657
- *The Nikkei Weekly* 1-800-322-1657
- *Outside* 1-800-678-1131
- PC Magazine 1-800-335-1195
- *PC Today* 1-800-544-1296
- *PC World* 1-800-825-7595
- *People* 1-800-541-1000
- *Premiere* 1-800-289-2489
- *Ranger Rick* 1-800-588-1650
- *Reader's Digest* 1-800-234-9000
- *Road & Track* 1-800-876-8316
- *Scientific America* 1-800-333-1199
- *Ski* 1-800-238-1616
- *Sports Illustrated* 1-800-541-1000
- *Time* 1-800-541-1000
- *Travel & Leisure* 1-800-888-8728
- *USA TODAY* 1-800-USA-0001
- *U.S. News & World Report* 1-800-544-9224
- *Vogue* 1-800-234-2347
- *The Wall Street Journal* 1-800-345-8502
- *Women's Sports & Fitness* 1-800-877-5280
- *Working Mother* 1-800-627-0690
- *Working Woman* 1-800-234-9675
- *Worth* 1-800-777-1851

For books that have been audio-produced:

Recorded Books, Inc. provides unabridged single-voice performances on book-packaged cassettes, featuring the very best books in- and out-of-print, available for both rental and purchase, by mail. For more information and a free catalog, call 1-800-638-1304.

Shopping by Television

Cable stations:
- QVC (Quality Value and Commitment)
- HSN (Home Shopping Network)

Shopping by Internet

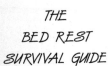
1. Go to one of the following search engines and type in your favorite retailer or mail-order company. Odds are they have an on-line site where you can either order products or a catalog.
   - www.yahoo.com
   - www.altavista.com
   - www.excite.com
   - www.askjeeves.com
   - www.jango.com
2. For books:
   - www.amazon.com
3. For travel:
   - www.thetrip.com
4. For children's entertainment:
   - www.bonus.com
5. For miscellaneous:
   - www.infospace.com
   - www.bigbook.com (white pages/telephone book)
   - www.bigyello.com (yellow pages/telephone book)
   - www.worldpages.com (international white, yellow, and blue (government) pages)

CHAPTER FIVE

Smart and Savory Picnics

*O*n bed rest, eating may be difficult at first. Your appetite may decrease, or you may feel like eating everything you can get your hands on (if this is so, it is probably better that your access to the refrigerator is limited). Constipation as well as complications with meal preparation add to the challenge. And, unfortunately, you will find that your reclining position makes it difficult to drink and eat certain foods.

My first attempts at drinking liquids were wet and frustrating (not only were the pillowcase and sheets uncomfortable, so was being dependent on someone else to clean them up). Discovering a lid-covered toddler cup was a lifesaver.

The first dinner wasn't much better. My favorite linguini swayed and sprayed marinara sauce everywhere! Clearly, the noodles were too stringy and the sauce too messy for my bedridden position. After a round of discussion, my husband and I agreed that the best choice for pasta à la bed rest would be penne or shells. A compact noodle holds the sauce and stays on the fork. The need for a bib became apparent! You will find, through trial and error, that certain foods work better than others. Remember, uncomplicated foods need not be unimaginative foods.

Eating well is crucial to your healing process and important for maintaining health. It is worth testing the waters to discover what appeals on a practical level and to your palate. I favored eating small meals five to six times a day. Eventually, eating will become manageable and more fun as you and your helpers learn the art and science of bedside picnicking. If you hire a home-care service to do your shopping, meal preparation and serving (Refer to Chapter 2, Immediate Preparation and the Supplies and Services Guide in Appendix E for more information on out-side services), communicate verbally and in written form how you prefer your meals. Being bedridden doesn't mean you can't enjoy your favorite foods at mealtime. In the next section on setup, supplies and many ideas, I suggest you cut out these pages for use by your meal provider.

There are, however, a few basic rules of thumb for dining à la bed rest.

Rule #1. Drink lots of liquids. Any physician will tell you that hydration is important for healing and sustaining healthy bodies. Dehydration can foster serious med-ical complications. It is strongly recommended that you drink at least eight glasses of water every day, even if getting up to use the toilet is forbidden or a hassle.

Rule #2. Choose foods high in vitamins and minerals, pro-viding the most nutrition for the calories. For build-ing strength in healing and for pregnancy, foods rich in iron, calcium, magnesium, zinc, and the B-vitamin folic acid are best.

Rule #3. Since constipation is a universal bed rest problem, fiber and fluids are more important than ever. Warm or hot drinks will help considerably.

Rule #4. Delegate. You have no choice. This will require clear communication of your needs and wants, how, when, and where you and/or others will dine (you may be delegating responsibility for others' meals, i.e. small children, kitchen-disabled spouses, elderly dependents). Some of your success in giving up control will depend on your care provider(s). Choose someone who is positive, accountable, and sensitive to your circumstances.

Helpful sources for the recommended nutrients:

- Fiber: whole-grain cereals and breads, fresh fruits and vegetables, legumes, dried beans and peas, wheat-bran and oat-bran products
- Fluids: six to eight glasses of water or other noncaloric caffeine-free beverages daily in addition to milk and juice
- Protein: lean meat, poultry, fish, eggs, beans, tofu, legumes, nuts, and nut butters
- Iron: lean red meats (beef, lamb, and pork), dark green leafy vegetables, canned sardines, fortified cereals and grain products—To enhance absorption of iron from non-meat sources, combine them with other foods high in vitamin C, such as lemon juice, tomatoes, oranges, and other citrus fruits and juices.
- Calcium: low-fat and reduced-fat milk products such as milk, cheese, yogurt, frozen yogurt and ice milk, broccoli and other dark green leafy vegetables, canned sardines and salmon (calcium comes from the edible bones)
- Folic Acid: oranges, orange juice, spinach, romaine lettuce, dark green leafy vegetables, beans, wheat germ, and nuts

The setup:

I found it helpful to have consistency in the way my foods were organized and set up around me. My husband developed a system for putting out my breakfast, lunch, and snacks. He did the same thing every day. Each morning, the foods that I had requested (a handwritten list for breakfast, lunch, and snacks), were placed on my breakfast tray or in the cooler. This routine made it manageable for my husband, and I, in turn, knew exactly what to expect. I could always count on the large hot water thermos so that there was always a choice between making hot tea, fresh brewed decaffeinated coffee, cocoa, or hot juice. My toddler cups were always clean and available for cold drinks. Spare water bottles, fresh ice in the cooler, and all of my snack bags were daily staples and always included on the picnic tray. With the gamut of choices provided, I thrived on our self-created self-serve routine. After a while, it was hard to imagine normal life without the bedside cooler, the plastic baggie salad bar, the hand wipes, and the dirty-dish container!

Supplies for picnics in bed:

- ❑ Lap tray
- ❑ Ice chest with the daily staples such as a water jug, ice packs or bagged ice, condiments—butter, mayonnaise, mustard, salad dressing, peanut butter—and snacks such as carrot sticks, apples, string cheese
- ❑ Water bottles, toddler tippy cups or cups with straws
- ❑ Utensils: fork, spoon, cutting knife, small to medium-size cutting board, plate, bowl—paper and plastic are easier if you are home alone for most of the day
- ❑ Snack bags with nonperishable foods—trail mix, dried fruit, bagels, sandwich bread, crackers (these should be refilled each morning)
- ❑ Salt and pepper shakers
- ❑ Dirty-dish container
- ❑ Bib
- ❑ Thermos or electric-coil water heater (must be connected to electrical outlet, which may require an extension cord)

❏ Small microwave
❏ Blender (optional—for liquid meals or if smoothies are your favorite!)

*Each day the utensils should be cleaned or replaced. All foods should be replenished. The thermos, bibs, water bottles, etc. should be emptied, rinsed, and dried for the next day of bed rest picnicking.

Menu Ideas

When you're faced with a situation like bed rest, it is easy to forget some of the most basic options for meals. In an attempt to remind you of the simple yet delicious choices, I have organized menus by meal (breakfast, snacks, lunch, and dinner). Additionally, I have included lists of foods by nutritional category, e.g. proteins, iron-rich foods, etc. My hope is that you and your helpers will use these ideas to produce nutritious and delicious meals. You will see that once the job of shopping and preparing your foods is done (thanks to a helping hand), you can easily enjoy your very own bed rest smorgasbord.

Breakfast:
Instant hot cereal packages
Cereal with yogurt and fruit
Cottage cheese with fruit
Granola
Kasha (pilaf for breakfast, lunch, or dinner—sodium- and cholesterol-free)
Soft- or hard-boiled, scrambled, or poached eggs with toast and fruit
Tender asparagus makes a natural, edible utensil. Delicious alongside a cooked egg, dunk it into egg yolk, stir, and eat.
Bagels and cream cheese, add lox, tomato, and onion, etc. if desired
Whole grain waffles with maple syrup, honey, or fruit

French toast with maple syrup, honey, or fruit
Cinnamon toast and applesauce
Fruit salad and toast
Muffin with fruit
Whole wheat scones (prebuy at favorite bakery and freeze in Ziploc bags)

Breakfast drinks are good sources of your daily fluid requirements. I recommend you start each day with hot tea, coffee, cocoa, hot juice, or warm milk. Thermoses, hot water coils, and microwaves are essential bed rest equipment for enjoying warm drinks throughout the entire day and evening. (More suggestions for a variety of fluids to follow.) Also, in an effort to maintain your daily nutritional requirements, add yogurt, cheese, fruits, veggies, meat, or fish to your breakfast whenever possible.

Easy-to-make and highly nutritious snacks

You may prefer to have four to six snacks during the day rather than a routine breakfast and lunch. This choice may in part depend on your kitchen help or your ability to organize and request what should be left on the bed during the time you are required to be self-sufficient. Finger foods should be just that. Awkward, sticky, soggy, or drippy foods have no place in bed. Energy bars may be the best solution for those of you whose resources are extremely limited.

Snack ideas:
Deviled eggs
Celery with peanut butter and raisins
Sliced carrots, celery, radishes, and green onions—keep fresh in cold water
Dips: humus, spinach/sour cream, cream cheese, peanut butter—many can be premade or bought as mixes that just need water
String cheese

Cheese and crackers

Sliced fruit: apple, pear, peach, orange, banana, melon, kiwi, avocado—Squeeze lemon over apple, avocado, banana, and pear so they don't brown.

Nuts and raisins

Dried fruits

Low-fat cereal bars

Mixed cereals (i.e. Wheat Chex, oat squares, pretzels)

Applesauce

Yogurt

Rice cakes—plain or with cream cheese, peanut butter, apple butter, etc.

Frozen fruit molds—cut up a variety of fruits, add lemonade or apple juice and freeze in an ice cube tray or any other mold.

Frozen yogurt—premix a container of yogurt, put in freezer, and enjoy a low-fat ice-yogurt treat (recommended: vanilla, coffee, and caramel yogurts)

Frozen grapes, bananas, kiwi

Cooked baby red potatoes

Sliced red pepper with cream-cheese spread or dip

Popcorn

Crunchy and cold pickles

Marinated black or green olives

Energy foods such as: Clif Bar, PowerBar, Stoker Bar, etc. are made from whole grains and fruit. They are rich in simple carbohydrates for quick energy, and complex carbohydrates for sustained energy. This is the easiest and healthiest way to refuel.

Lunch:

Always balance your meal with a drink, fruit, protein, and vegetable.

Soup in a thermos with baguette and cheese

Instant soup, preferably a brand that contains no preservatives and is low in sodium *squeeze lemon into hot or cold soups to intensify the flavor

Bagel and cream cheese—add lox, salami, etc.

Fresh fruit salad—serve with yogurt or cottage cheese

Salad bar—mix together vegetables, fruit, cheese, raisins, nuts

Peanut butter-and-jelly sandwich

Tuna salad sandwich

Egg salad sandwich

Chicken or turkey salad sandwich

Ham-and-cheese sandwich

Grilled cheese sandwich

Pita with humus or seafood salad, chicken salad, egg salad, etc.

Pizza—frozen, premade dough for make-your-own

Quesadilla

Deli meats with pickles and cheese

Dry salami and cheese on crackers

Baked potato

Apple chunks with ham

Swiss cheese cubes and ham cubes on a skewer or toothpick to eat

Beef and turkey jerky

Steamed (crisp) vegetables: broccoli, artichoke, beets, carrots, corn on the cob

Dinner leftovers

Keep a jar of chutney, jam, olive or basil pesto in your cooler and try it on roast meat sandwiches, hot or cold, or with cheese and crackers.

Dinner:

In the United States, dinner is traditionally the largest meal of the day and the more "official" meal when family and friends eat together and socialize.

On bed rest, it is best to keep dinners simple, just like your other meals. Whoever is doing the cooking should focus on nutritious low-fat foods as well as satisfying the "customer"—YOU! If your partner is cooking, try to keep the whole situation in perspective. For instance, he or she may not be used to cooking. The effort required may be more than you can imagine. They may feel more like spending time with you than fussing in the kitchen. The result may be meals that aren't very good. Try to be patient. Encourage your helpers and emphasize simplicity with fresh fruits and veggies, whole grains with your favorite dairy products. This way, no one can go wrong.

The following ideas for meal preparation are for you and your cooking help. These suggestions are from family and friends who successfully managed to keep someone well fed during bed rest.

1. Freeze ahead! Label everything beforehand and, whenever possible, obtain defrosting and cooking instructions from the original chef. You can write directly on aluminum foil with a permanent marker.

2. Using two or three master recipes, variations from the same theme can be created. For example, if someone makes a large batch of tomato sauce, you can store it in the freezer for pasta sauce, lasagna, chili, pizza, etc. If a large amount of chicken is cooked, debone it, divide the meat, and save for making chicken pot pie, chicken enchiladas, chicken stew, chicken soup, chicken divan, etc.

3. Bake one large turkey or ham. Use the leftovers. Afterward, a hearty soup can be made from the remaining bone.

4. Double and triple casserole ingredients. Cook and serve one now, freeze the rest.

5. Prepare large soups and stews. Freeze the extra. Good for simple entertaining of visitors.

6. Steam vegetables slightly (crisp) and serve throughout the week.

7. It's worth it to spend the time making large fresh fruit salads that can be served throughout the week.

8. If someone likes to bake, have them bake extra amounts to be frozen and enjoyed over time.

THE BASIC DINNER FORMULA:

> **Salad + Main Course + Bread/Rice + Dessert (optional) = Dinner**

Salad ideas:
1. Mixed greens with onions, avocado, tomato, and carrots
2. Romaine lettuce with parmesan cheese, croutons, and Caesar dressing
3. Spinach, red onion, dried cranberries, goat cheese, roasted pinenuts, and rice vinegar/oil dressing
4. Carrot salad with raisins, pineapples, mayonnaise, or yogurt dressing
5. Butter lettuce with tangerines, green onions, and oil/vinegar dressing
6. Greek salad with feta cheese, olives, peppers, and lettuce

Main course ideas:
1. Pasta with sauce: tomato, pesto, alfredo, clams
2. Sliced ham
3. Sliced turkey
4. Lasagna
5. Stir-fried vegetables—add sauces to give it an ethnic flavoring/Indian curry, Chinese sesame oil, oyster sauce, Thai spices, etc.
6. Hearty soups and stews
7. Baked potato stuffed with cheese, vegetables, meats
8. Fish
9. Sausages
10. Meat: pork chops, lamb chops, steaks, chicken, veal
11. Pizza—premade crusts make this very easy; try a variety

of toppings such as goat cheese, green onions, sausage, eggplant, sun-dried tomatoes, etc.

12. Chicken, turkey, or vegetable pot pie
13. Meat loaf
14. Burritos: bean-and-cheese, chicken, pork, beef, steak

Breads/rice:

1. Bread, breadsticks, crackers, pita, bagels
2. Focaccia
3. Rice
4. Potato: boiled, mashed, baked, french fries, etc.
5. Risotto
6. Bulgur
7. Polenta
8. Couscous

Dessert (optional):

1. Fruit
2. Tapioca or pudding cups
3. Sorbet—bars or scooped in a dish
4. Ice Cream—bars or scooped in a dish
5. Freshly baked goods, e.g. brownies, lemon squares, cookies, pie, etc.

ALTERNATIVES TO HOME COOKING:

There will be many times while you're on bed rest when either no one is available or no one feels like cooking. Everyone needs a break. There will also be times when someone, whether it's you, your partner, your child, or a visiting friend has an urge for takeout. There is no better time than during this temporary period of confinement to take advantage of delivery services.

You can be the gatherer of takeout menus, phone numbers for home-cooking services, restaurants that offer a delivery service. If you're at a loss, check with local restaurants, schools, hospitals, and the Yellow Pages for their local resources. Depending on where you live, there are many ethnic choices available for your palate!

- Chinese
- Italian
- Pizza
- Mexican
- Mediterranean/Greek
- French
- American delicatessen
- Japanese/sushi
- Indian
- California cuisine
- Contemporary American
- Vietnamese
- Cambodian
- Ethiopian
- Seafood
- Thai
- Spanish

(Refer to Appendix E—Home Services and Supply Sources for meal providers.)

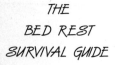
An Important Word on Liquids

You cannot drink enough! Every chance you can get, drink a glass of water. Virtually every cell in the body needs water to survive. Water transports nutrients to all parts of the body via the blood. It also serves as the medium for thousands of life-supporting chemical reactions constantly taking place in our bodies.

When I was on bed rest, I made a vow. Every time I went to the bathroom, got off the telephone, started a new activity, or ate something, I drank a glass of water. I encourage you to do the same.

Some favorite sources of fluid are:
1. Cold water
2. Mineral water (seltzer)

3. Warm apple juice with cinnamon stick (extra source of vitamin C)
4. Juice in a box (preferably 100% juice)
5. Lemonade
6. Tomato juice
7. Prune juice
8. Juice-flavored ice cubes
9. Fruit popsicles
10. Low-fat or nonfat milk
11. Caffeine-free tea and coffee
12. Fruit shake—Blend together juice, banana or melon, yogurt, and ice cubes. Freeze it the night before and let it thaw in your ice chest during the day. Frozen fruit and milk blended together works very well.

Try to eliminate high-sugar drinks like sodas. Many are filled with caffeine, sugar, and saccharin. These substances may reduce your ability to feel well and focus on healing.

NUTRITIONAL SAMPLERS:

PROTEINS
low-fat milk
milk shakes
low-fat or nonfat yogurt
frozen yogurt (freeze regular yogurt)
ice milk
buttermilk

✳

cheese cubes
string cheese
grated cheese
parmesan
bags of crumbled blue, feta, pot or farmer's cheese

✳

hard-boiled or soft-boiled egg
tofu
textured vegetable protein

✳

nuts and seeds
wheat germ

✳

freshwater fish
seafood
chicken
turkey
beef
lamb
pork
veal

✳

legumes
peas
beans
lentils

VITAMIN C FOODS:
fruit and vegetable juices
orange
mango
papaya
apricots
cantaloupe
strawberries
blackberries
raspberries
blueberries
figs
tomatoes

cabbage
broccoli
green pepper
cauliflower
sweet potato
kale
kohlrabi
spinach

CALCIUM-RICH FOODS:
low-fat or nonfat milk
low-fat buttermilk
evaporated skim or low-fat milk
low-fat cottage cheese
Cheddar or Swiss cheese
low-fat or nonfat yogurt
nonfat dry milk
orange juice
almonds
filberts
peanuts
dried fruit (sulfur-free)
canned salmon with bones
canned sardines with bones
sesame seeds
soy milk and protein
dark leafy greens
broccoli
figs
cooked beans

IRON-RICH FOODS:
dried fruit (sulfur-free is best)
beef
duck
liver
oysters (don't eat raw)

sardines
potatoes in their skin
spinach
seaweed
legumes (green peas and chickpeas, kidney and lima beans, lentils)
soybeans and soy products
blackstrap molasses
carob flour and carob powder

VEGETABLES:
asparagus
green beans
sugar snap peas
jicama
red, yellow, green bell peppers
cucumbers
brussel sprouts
mushrooms
okra
zucchini
broccoli
carrots
corn
beets
artichokes
celery
arugula
onion

CHAPTER SIX

Sexuality and Bed Rest

As difficult as bed rest is for you, it is also a difficult time for those close to you. It is hard for partners, children, and extended family to see a loved one challenged by medical problems. With all of the issues to confront owing to the extreme physical limitations and change of lifestyle, the display of love and affection between you and others may get forgotten.

All people require attention and care. It is an aspect of human sexuality. While you are on bed rest—alone, still, and experiencing a wide range of emotions—human connections take on a greater significance. You may find that, in unique ways, bed rest offers opportunities to grow very close to important people in your life.

For most, the experience of bed rest is a vulnerable time, physically and socially. The situation takes you out of your ordinary lifestyle and exposes the deep need we have to receive and to give. Bed rest can introduce a whole new dynamic in relationships and can foster new ways of communication: you may be receiving and giving more emotional support and physical affection than you're used to; you may begin to experience deeper connections with certain people in your life; gestures from others may seem almost exaggerated; and you may even feel a flair of romance, passion, or ecstasy within your platonic relationships. From personal experience as well as from the many bed rest stories I've heard, friendships and romance during bed rest seem to be enhanced! At a time when feelings of isolation and confinement abound, the powers of affection and intimate connection revive the soul. There is nothing more valuable for healing the mind and body. True healing has more to do with listening and loving than with trying to fix people.

I shall always remember the love and good care I received throughout my three months on bed rest. It came in many different forms. I absorbed all of it like a sponge!

What seemed especially meaningful was the love and positive reinforcement I received from my husband. And I know he appreciated my affectionate gestures in return. Together, we discovered wonderful ways of being close. My irritable uterus, the reason for my bed rest, prohibited sexual play of any kind. At first we were uneasy about any kind of touching. Gradually, we discovered the joy of gentle stroking, especially to our foreheads and forearms. These simple pleasures, in addition to just spending quality time together, was the most nurturing of all. Our limitations ultimately became a source of emotional and physical intimacy throughout my three months of stillness. Together, our hearts did a lot of dancing!

Family and friends had differing ways of expressing their love and concern. The circumstances of bed rest seemed to have infused my surroundings with a virginlike sensitivity and vulnerability. All of my exchanges with people shifted from the everyday lightweight and friendly manner to a deep, more personal and meaningful connection. What transpired was a new level of caring and loving that I had not previously shared with various people in my life. My bed rest experience offered great insights into the larger heart of humanity, and I grew to appreciate and value the meaning of compassion.

There really is nothing like kind and loving relationships. When you have this in your life, especially when you're bedridden, it provides you with support and reinforcement. It instills you with a feeling of confidence and peace.

My bed rest experience turned out to be a personal sanctuary in my life that drew near to me many generous people in my life. It was a safe haven where my health and hope were nourished.

I deeply believe that bed rest can offer all relationships—including kinships with animals—a deeper intimacy that might not otherwise occur.

EXERCISES TO IMPROVE INTIMACY

Identification and Acknowledgment

For encouraging and creating more open and loving relationships, try to answer these two questions daily as an affirmation or in a journal.

- What would help me to feel good right now?
- What do I think would help make others in my life feel good?

Suggestions for Enhancing Intimacy

The following are aspects of intimacy that will require your special attention during bedrest:

Verbal affection:
words of encouragement
words of appreciation
validation
acknowledgment
frequent and consistent communication
asking questions with genuine interest

Physical affection:
Being touched and held is a very basic human need. Studies have shown that infants without frequent and direct contact have delayed development. Recent studies show the importance of

touch and its contribution to personal fortification in all ages. For instance, massage is shown to be effective against depression and hypertension. Cuddling and sleeping skin-to-skin can do everything from lowering blood pressure to strengthening the immune system. Skin is considered to be the largest sex organ. There is great power in soft, gentle, loving touching.

- Ways to be close with friends: holding hands, an arm easily thrown around the shoulder, hugs, rubbing necks, arms, shoulders, head, hands, and feet. *Bed rest examples*: While I was on bed rest, a friend asked me if it would feel good if she brushed my hair. We talked and she brushed for a wonderful two-hour visit! A work associate came to visit and held my hand the minute she saw me. Soon I realized she was doing acupressure on my hand. I felt immeasurably better because of her genuine concern and interest which came through in this very special way. Another friend, a professional masseuse, came to visit once a week. We talked while she worked on my feet. The amount of stress buildup in feet is extraordinary, even if you're lying down all the time! Foot and hand massages are another wonderful way to rejuvenate and great for enhancing friendships.
- For intimate exchanges with your partner, especially when abstention from intercourse is required, try the following: cuddling, long soulful kisses, hugging, holding hands, body massage. You may want to obtain the book *Romantic Massage,* by Anne Kent Rush (1996).
- Arrange romantic time alone with your partner: a candlelit dinner, schedule a date to watch a special video, listen to music, read together.
- Sexual intimacy*: erotic cuddling, kissing, massaging, masturbation. Penetration must be medically approved. Always proceed with caution if there is the slightest chance of causing further medical risk.

*Consult with your physician, as arousal of any form may cause further medical complications.

Gentle displays of affection:

- Reading together.
- Listening: This simple act can greatly improve communication and mean a tremendous amount to someone who feels the need to be heard. It may not always be the bedridden person who needs the ear.
- Breathing together: The way we breathe can influence our state of mind. Breathing is important not just for thriving physically but mentally and emotionally as well. Like anything else that is being shared, breathing with someone can bring quiet understanding and warmth between two people or a group of friends. When my contractions would flare up at night, my husband would calm me by lying close to me and guiding me in breathing. We would breathe together for as long as it took me to feel that my body was calm and the contractions had ceased. Some hints: exhaling more slowly than we inhale calms the mind. Inhaling more slowly than we exhale energizes it. Balancing two breaths brings a calm to the body.
- Exchanging love poems, notes of appreciation, drawings, simple gifts. One Sunday afternoon, my two-year-old niece came to visit. She insisted on getting into bed with me, shoes and all. She had a surprise gift for me and didn't want anyone else to see it. Way under the sheets, she gave me a colorful crayon drawing on a little piece of scrap paper. It was an intimate moment for both of us, and a meaningful gesture that made me feel loved.

For Valentine's Day, I cut out and pasted homemade cards. It was great fun to feel like a child again. I was able to say hello and thank you to all the neighbors, friends, work associates, and family members who had been helping me so much.

Another time, my husband arrived home later than usual from work. At first I was upset because he knew my day had been especially hard. He greeted me with a kiss and a crumpled paper bag. In the package was a soft flannel nightgown with

two holes in the front. It was for nursing our baby! I really appreciated this thoughtful and practical gift. I returned the thoughtful gesture with a handmade thank-you card that I put under his
pillow that night.

CHAPTER SEVEN

✗

You're Not Alone

*E*veryone on bed rest has his or her own unique adventure and yet, as you will see by the following adventures, you're not alone. The good news is that all of us who have experienced the epic journey through bed rest have now traveled way beyond our horizontal stories.

Kimberly (36 years old)

Eleven years ago I was bedridden with my first pregnancy. After eight days of trying to stop labor Alex, my son, was born at twenty-eight weeks gestation. He weighed only two pounds. Because of complications, he spent the next seven months in the intensive care unit. While he grew to become strong and healthy, he was left with a lifetime disability, mild cerebral palsy. During my next pregnancy, I was extremely cautious, as I had preeclampsia. Ben, my second child, was born two weeks early.

With my third pregnancy I went into preterm labor more than three months before my due date. As a result, I spent four months on strict bed rest. Faced again with the possibility of a premature birth, I fully accepted the bed rest requirement.

First, I called my mother on the East Coast and asked her to come stay with us until we found some help. At the time, Ben was four years old and had just started kindergarten and Alex, seven, was in third grade. My mother stayed with us for a month.

My friends and neighbors were incredible! Food arrived at our home every night. Dinner deliveries continued through the first month after the baby's birth. My friends brought everything: salad, main course, bread, dessert. We got to the point where we had too much food, so one of my friends took over the scheduling and arranged for deliveries on Mondays, Wednesdays, and Fridays.

Neighbors and friends took my kids to school, drove me to the doctor's, called all the time, and brought me books. When everyone was at school or work, I spent a lot of time listening to National Public Radio. I brought myself up-to-date with current events and politics. I especially enjoyed defending various controversial issues on the show, *Talk of the Nation.*

A friend who lived across the street was also pregnant. She wanted to learn how to knit, so every day, I gave her a knitting lesson while we talked.

Having a kindergartner meant I had company every afternoon. Ben would climb into bed with me. We'd read and play games. When Alex arrived home, we'd read and play some more and I'd help him with board games.

I tried very hard to manage the stress level of the whole family. I organized everyone's life very carefully. I didn't want my bed rest to create more of a burden for my husband and children. I tried to keep myself steady as well. I listened to tapes, read spiritual books, and studied Italian. When my children got upset about my situation, I allowed them to stay home with me so they could feel as close to me as they needed to be. When my husband wanted to be intimate, I stayed very accessible without ever risking my own health. I opened up completely to my family, and I was able to be very generous with my affection.

Once I knew I could control the labor by staying off my feet and I was clear about my symptoms, I focused on keeping myself hydrated and watching my blood pressure. I was very careful about adhering to my bed rest requirements. I kept reminding myself about my goal of carrying my baby to full term and then bringing it home with me.

The inconvenience and restrictions of bed rest are nothing compared to the heartache of having an infant spend months in the hospital. This is the most important message I could ever pass on to other pregnant women. When you're solely responsible for the health of your baby, there's no choice in the matter. A mother can follow bed rest so much easier than an infant can endure intensive care. Although my doctor told me I could get up toward the end of my term, I didn't. To me, it wasn't worth the risk. I knew the best possibility for my child was to remain and fully develop within my uterus for the full term. I have learned the alternative.

Larry (45 years old)

My lifetime career in law enforcement ended one day four years ago after a routine physical. The doctor found extensive cancer in my pancreas. With no other choice but certain death, I agreed to immediate surgery, previously one of my greatest fears.

My story is somewhat of a miracle. And yet, I never would have guessed the power of the mind and spirit. I am presently back at work and in full remission. Reflecting back, however, it was the potency of family love, friendships, and my own self-discovery that pulled me through. I was never a big communicator at home. While I had a lot going on in my head, it usually churned away inside of me and spilled out at work: meetings, training sessions, etc. From the time I learned of my illness through the early days of recovery, I experienced significant personal shift. I began reaching out. To everyone. I let my family know how much I loved them. They showered me with the deepest love a man can know. People from work came to visit me, and despite the obvious shock and despair, a lot of love and prayers were exchanged. Reflecting back, the power of love and self-discovery is what pulled me through this trauma.

Once I began embracing the things I loved in life, I felt my health begin to improve. Bed rest afforded me the time to empower myself. The love from family and friends, the reward of activities that brought me deep personal joy, and the time to realize and obtain the little things that made me feel special each day opened my way for successful healing.

The most profound revelation I gained from my two months on bed rest is that every individual has the ability to go way beyond his or her status quo. Prior to my bed rest experience, I was not in touch with my whole self. I spent little or no time thinking about the meaning of relationships or the value of love. Although I am a sensitive person, I am very practical and lived my life that way. I had no idea who I really was deep inside. I didn't know I was capable of true feelings and spiritual thoughts. My experience on bed rest opened up another dimension of who I am. I'm a bigger person, and I experience more from everyday interactions and activity than I did before my days healing in bed. I learned something very important about all people. Whether you're old or young, in school or at work, on a soccer field or in bed for months, there is a whole other level of potential within ready to be tapped.

Margaret (48 years old)

Several years ago, when I was in my late twenties, my podiatrist recommended foot surgery for a problem that had been bothering me for almost a decade. I was, at the time, almost crippled. Walking was painful, and running, which had been my almost-profession for several years, was becoming impossible. The bunions on my feet had become so large and so arthritic, that I had to cut holes in the front corner of my shoes in order to wear anything comfortably on my feet. Needless to say, I looked like an orphan. So, I had surgery. And, since I was used to being independent and very resourceful, I imagined that after the initial shock to my body from surgery, I would be able to take care of myself and would bounce back quite soon.

But that was not the script. I was bedridden for much longer than my strong-willed mind would have liked to imagine, and it was an enormous adjustment to depend on other people to take care of even my most basic needs. I could only crawl, which I found quite humorous, and thought it was a metaphor for a psyche who, in its deepest recesses, would never have allowed myself to be seen that way. It was a lesson in humility and a short detention for my spiraling need to never, I repeat, never need help.

As hard as it was for me to say, I needed other people. I think, they enjoyed and appreciated the part of me that finally had to admit it and accept their generosity. They had a useful place in my life, and I realized, perhaps for the first time, how much we all crave to be useful to one another. It is often said that you learn lessons the hard way and I learned a very valuable lesson: not only is it okay to be appropriately needy, but other people are often looking for ways to fit into your life. They want to help, take care, give, offer comfort, or just simply make a very gentle difference in your life. It makes a difference in their lives.

So even though my feet have stopped hurting, I often ask for help—a little assistance, a short ride somewhere, a cup of sugar, or a borrowed book. I think I'm better off for it.

Ginger (38 years old)

I was first diagnosed as a DES daughter when I was seventeen. I was told at the time that I had a "hood" on my cervix (that was cauterized off), but that there were no other symptoms of DES exposure that I should be concerned about. When I asked about having children in the future, the physician said no problem.

My husband and I learned about our first pregnancy in January 1986. I was twenty-eight. I immediately found a physician to confirm the pregnancy and the hopes and dreams began immediately. On my third prenatal visit, one of the older members of the OB-Gyn team examined me for the first time and asked me if I had been pregnant before. I said no. His response to me was, "Well, you had better chalk this pregnancy up to history, as you will never carry this baby to term. You don't have a cervix that is worth mentioning." I was devastated and VERY frightened, as I wasn't really sure what a cervix was for, but it obviously was necessary for pregnancy. I went home and immediately found another OB. This doctor was very supportive and told me to take it easy, no vacuuming, lifting, and that it would probably be a good idea not to have any sex either.

We carried on in a fragile state for the next couple of months. I quit my job and "hung around the house." I couldn't wait to go out and buy my first maternity outfit. Ironically the day that I bought my first maternity dress was the day that my cervix started to dilate. It was mid-May. The doctor put me on bed rest immediately and said to keep my feet higher than my heart. I stayed that way for six days. At my next appointment it was decided that I needed to go to Sacramento to the perinatal specialists. Upon my arrival, I went into labor. I was rushed to the local hospital and put in a Trendelunberg position, a bed position where the head is kept lower than the feet. At this point my doctor decided that a vaginal cerclage, a sewn stitch to keep the cervix closed, wouldn't hold, and they began thinking about an abdominal cerclage. I was then pumped full of drugs—terbutaline was the favorite—and given a bedpan. I remember thinking "How is this going to work if I am on my head?"

The labor stopped thanks to the drugs, and luckily they let me put the bed in a normal position for my toileting needs. I ate and slept and received visitors in the Trendelenburg position for the next four weeks. The hospital became a very safe place. My mother put her life on hold, much to my father's chagrin, and stayed by my bed from sunup to sundown each and every day. It was an incredible time for the two of us. She had taken a drug, DES, to save her pregnancy, which in turn had resulted in putting me in a position that was identical. Now I was taking any drug they gave me to save my baby.

After everything calmed down, it was decided that I could return home to Chico (two hours away) and await the arrival of the baby. The second day home, I began leaking amniotic fluid, which was not a good sign. I knew the baby was only twenty-five weeks along at best. Back down to Sacramento we went. My old room was still available, and I felt relieved to be back with my friends, back on my head, and safe. Four days later my water broke. We were at 26 ½ to 27 weeks. That was the big goal they kept giving me, and we achieved it. My doctor announced that there was going to be a birthday. My family, friends, and I were thrilled! There was true joy on all of our faces and the staff did an incredible job of "playing along" with the happy occasion, never letting on that they knew what a twenty-seven-week-old baby meant. We delivered a two pound, five ounce son hours later by C-section, again an unpleasant experience due to the epidural. We named him James Peter and felt the incredible joy of parenthood immediately.

Our perception continued to be that we had delivered a perfectly healthy baby. They had said two pounds was good, we gave them two pounds, five ounces! They said 26 weeks was good, we gave them 27! Within the hour we were told that the baby's lungs had collapsed and that he had a hemorrhage on his brain. It was only a short time later that a doctor I did not know walked in, looked at Jim and me and said the words that I will never forget, "Your baby is dead."

My friends at the hospital taught us how to deal with the grief. We slowly returned to "real life" and began making plans for our next baby. We scheduled our next surgery for the abdominal cerclage the following January. It was felt that performing the surgery in a nonpregnant state might give the doctors a better chance of placing the cerclage in a more secure way. Abdominal cerclages were supposed to be a one-time surgery. My previous one had ruptured and had to be removed during the C-section. The second cerclage was put in January of 1987.

I found out I was pregnant again in August of 1987. I was incredibly calm about this second pregnancy and had a gut feeling that we were going to be OK. The doctors were very cautious in their care, and kept making reference to the fact that we now had a "history." I was put on strict bed rest at approximately 18 weeks. I had been using progesterone suppositories since about three months and had been restricting my activities prior to the bed rest. They originally said bed rest meant only getting up to go to the bathroom. I begged for a shower a day if I promised to sit down during the shower. They gave me that one. I remember buying a small Rubbermaid stool because it was wide enough to be comfortable. My mother-in-law came from Vermont and moved in with us for the last three months of the pregnancy. I remember feeling very Zen about this bed rest stint. I initially thought about learning a new language, books I wanted to read, old movies I wanted to see, etc. The most memorable experiences about that bed rest term were the visits from a friend, on a weekly basis, who would bring lunch and a movie. I also spent hours looking up at our dome ceiling while I counted knotholes. I couldn't read, as my mind would wander from the book. I didn't watch television. I didn't knit, didn't learn a foreign language either. My only attention seemed to be on making that baby. It was a very strange time. I do remember wishing a couple of times that my mother-in-law would fly back to Vermont!

We set up a queen-size mattress in the living room. In the morning I would shower, dress, eat, and move to the living room. I didn't return to the bedroom until it was time to go to bed. I found this to be crucial to my mental health, and it also helped my husband as well. My peace of mind regarding this pregnancy also came from my use of a Tokos home monitor. This device would read my uterine activity for two one-hour sessions a day. A nurse would call and ask me to send the information over the phone lines. They would read the strips and let me know if I had any activity. Whenever I felt nervous or unsure about my activity, I could put the monitor on and call in my strip, anytime of night or day. This was a great way to keep my stress level from getting too high. There was only one time when the strip was overly active. I was told to lie on my left side and drink a lot of water. I also had a prescription of terbutaline as a backup if needed. The daily contact with the staff at Tokos was imperative to my daily routine. They were just a phone call away. I continued to be monitored by the perinatal specialists in Sacramento.

We didn't have any "hairy" moments during this pregnancy. At 37 weeks, I began to have some pain at the site of the cerclage that was reminiscent of my previous pain when my cerclage was rupturing. I phoned Sacramento, and they said to come down right away. Some urgency returned. I could not be allowed to go into labor because of the cerclage and the vertical incision that had been made in my uterus when I delivered James Peter.

My daughter Chalen was born at 37 weeks. She was six pounds, nine ounces. And nineteen inches long. The cerclage had ruptured and had to be removed again. Chalen was truly my miracle baby. I had a strong feeling that she had been given to me by James Peter. I continue to view him as my angel who paid me a brief visit. Chalen was a gift from him. During her first year of life, I experienced an overwhelming fear of losing her. I was always afraid that something was going to happen to her, that I would lose her any moment. Though I recognized it stemmed from my prior loss and difficulty, I couldn't shake it. Chalen was our life!

We ended up moving back to Vermont four years later. I had just finished graduate school and was hired as a speech-language pathologist in Stowe, Vermont. Chalen, Jim, and I were getting used to a new life when we discovered that we were pregnant again. This was a total surprise, as we were just getting used to the idea of having only one child. I was petrified. I had just taken a new job, and I knew what my pregnancies entailed. I immediately called my perinatologist in California. I needed to know if I was tempting fate by asking for another child. His answer was no.

We began the process again. I went in for surgery at 12 weeks for my third cerclage. This time I insisted on a spinal for this surgery, as I had had such bad luck with epidurals. The surgery was a success. I recovered well and went back to work for four weeks before being placed once again on strict bed rest. We were a little smarter this time, and I realized that I needed to be "organized." I didn't need to do this all alone, and I asked for help. I hired a house cleaner just to come in and do the kitchen and bathroom. I asked Jim to get a firm foam mattress for the den, and I ordered a body pillow. I asked the doctor to order the Tokos program again. There was a slight argument about this, but I won! I knew that the monitoring program was crucial to my peace of mind. We set up a TV tray with all my "items" for the day on it. I made sure that my "daytime area" was in a strategic place in the house. I could see the front door from my bed as well as a great picture window with a view. A window is really important as it's a view to the outside world.

My husband was in between jobs so he was able to help out during the day. As it was the third time we had done this, everyone was a little more calm in their approach to bed rest. I started hooking a Persian-style rug, which was a great time passer. We got satellite television, which meant that I could watch all the old movies. We already had a success story, so we knew that this was a matter of trying to pass the time.

This was the pregnancy that I actually had cravings. I craved candy . . . chewy fruit types. This is what I would ask people to bring if they offered. I found I moved around the house this time a little more. I would have different places to go during different times. We used a recliner for the living room. This helped when visitors came. I wasn't "on the floor," which was more comfortable for the visitor. I found that having an ironing board next to my bed was also really helpful. The ironing board made a great adjustable table. I could lower it enough to use it in bed, and it was long enough to hold a myriad of stuff. We found the cheaper models were too flimsy. It was worth it to get a good sturdy model. A silly little pick-me-up was wearing funky socks. Because I was around the house all day, I tended to live in sweats and my husband's shirts, so the socks were my own statement. I also painted my nails a lot. It would make me feel like I was doing something.

I actually started to get bedsores at one point. We purchased an eggcrate mattress from a medical supply store. This was very helpful, and we changed its location every day and at night. Jim and I decided that a trip out of the house once in a while was an OK thing. It made a world of difference in my attitude. We would put the seats down and throw the body pillow in the car and off we would go.

I kept a calendar near my daytime area and would cross off each day before going to bed each night. Each month I would come up with a different symbol to be drawn on each space. I think it was pregnant bellies the first month, stars and moons the second, and baby bottles the third.

At 36 weeks, I began to feel the twinges of labor. We called the doctors, and they said to come in for an ultrasound. After my examination, it was determined that I should have an amnio to see if the baby's lungs were developed. The amnio came back fine, and the decision was made to deliver the baby instead of getting into a trauma situation. We set up the surgery for the next morning. We were concerned that there would be complications due to the scar tissue from previous surgeries, and asked the perinatologist to perform the surgery as opposed to a resident. The physician agreed. This C-section would be my sixth abdominal surgery.

Unfortunately, a resident performed the surgery and ended up nicking my bowel. Because the surgery became complicated, they went into medical mode. They delivered my son Peter, six pounds, nine ounces, nineteen inches long (exactly the same as his sister!). They forgot to include me in the birth, however, and I remember having to ask what the baby was, if he was OK, etc.

The hospital ended up discharging Peter while I was still in the hospital. Insurance reasons. I was devastated. We were able to figure out a way to keep Peter with me after he was discharged from the hospital. Two weeks after delivery we arrived home.

There isn't a day that goes by that I don't look at my children and think about how lucky I am to have them. I appreciate them so much! These days I look back on my bed rest experiences with mixed feelings. I miss the structure of those days. I always knew what to expect. I wouldn't hesitate encouraging anyone to make bed rest a positive experience. It's such a small price to pay for such an incredible outcome. My little motto that also helped me was "Patience is a virtue." I often think that bed rest and the difficulties we encountered with our children means that our payback is down the road—perhaps when our children are in their teens they won't talk back to their mother!!!

Yvette (36 years old)

On one of those fantastic midmorning visits to my OB-Gyn for our seven-month pregnancy check, my anticipated summer plans took a turn we didn't expect. My husband and I had been enjoying this pregnancy very much. It was our first together. My daughter from another marriage was six years old at the time, and very much the center of our lives. Gideon and I had been trying to get pregnant for four out of the five years we had been married. Unfortunately, I had been struggling with chronic fatigue syndrome, and our chances for success looked slim. Now, we felt blessed to know we were on our way to having it all!

The baby dropped so low and moved into position so prematurely that it put tremendous pressure on my lower organs and back. My doctor feared the blood supply to the placenta would be impacted by this position and that premature labor might be a possibility. I experienced early contractions at six months and had severe sciatica during the fourth and fifth months. Whether the doctor had ordered bed rest or not, I would have put myself on it. My legs and hips felt locked around my tightened and enormous uterus. There was no question my body needed to be reclining.

My husband was fantastic. He saw the writing on the wall as far as my limitations were concerned, and he took on dual roles.

We were not in a financial position to hire someone to take on my workload around the house. Gideon immediately organized a meeting to discuss the situation with everyone at his office, and within two days he had created a home office. Throughout my two months on bed rest, he did all the cooking, car pooling, dishes, etc. We were able to hire someone to come in once a week to do general cleaning and laundry.

Luckily, the timing of all of this didn't present a problem for my work. I'm a teacher, and I'd just finished the school year. I had, however, looked forward to spending quality time with my daughter during the summer months, when we were both out of school. I had anticipated this with so much pleasure, a last summer alone with my daughter. I knew life would never be quite the same once the new baby was born.

I missed sexual intimacy with my husband. We did a lot of cuddling. Gideon spent a lot of time massaging my back and rubbing my belly. It was so sweet, I will never forget this part of my bed rest.

I never really had a routine while on bed rest. I wanted to stay flexible. It was summer, I had just finished the school year, and, when the family was around, my first desire was to spend my time with them. We have always had a family tradition of hanging out talking and reading out loud to each other. As soon as I was bedridden, my daughter took it upon herself to set up a couch, cot, bed, or recliner in each room. Nothing would hold us back from traveling around the house to hang out, read together, and talk. In my bedridden state, I felt like a bird moving from one tree perch to another. After hours of lying in one spot, it felt good to move on to the next place.

I spent a lot of time speaking with friends on the telephone. They called to cheer me although I was in good spirits most of the time just knowing I was preparing to give birth. I read magazines. I listened to music more than usual, and, thanks to my daughter's portable piano, I practiced scales. We also had some paints and blank canvases in a closet. My daughter and I created some beautifully collaborated artwork that we have proudly framed in our new home. My favorite activity was knitting a blanket for the baby with small needles.

I had gestational diabetes, so my diet was very restricted and regimented. I found out I had gestational diabetes when I had the standard prenatal glucose test. For three months I had to draw blood from my fingers four times a day to moderate my glucose level. I took a urine sample daily to check for ketones, a type of insulin analysis. I kept a diary of everything I ate, drank, chewed, and swallowed. I was committed to only eating high-protein foods and carbohydrates. I could have absolutely no sweets, which meant giving up my big pregnancy craving. This was just a simple drink, a Snapple, but it was forbidden. My big treat was takeout Chinese or Thai food. Mostly, I ate chicken, fish, cheese (I had to be careful because I didn't want to gain too much weight), and vegetables. The dietary guide that I followed closely involved three snacks in addition to regular meals, something which was new for me. I was willing to do anything to stay healthy. My husband was a great source of encouragement. He always said, "This kind of diet will surely produce an exceptionally beautiful baby!"

I also drank a lot of Celestial Seasonings iced tea. Not only was it important for me to keep up my liquids, it was a very hot and beautiful summer. For me, this was like salt on a wound—the wound being my desire to be outdoors playing with my daughter. We lived in a home that had no outdoor sitting or play area. (It was a rental while we were rebuilding our home that was burned in one of the huge California wildfires.) I was not a happy camper, but tried to make the best of it. We kept all of the windows open, and fresh air breezed through. With cots and mattresses in every room, I literally followed the sun, and, whenever I could, I chose to lie like a kitty cat in a long stream of sunlight. This helped my moods a lot!

Holly (46 years old)

I am a doctor who is heading into my fourth year of bed rest. My husband, six-year-old son, and four-and-a-half-year-old daughter had taken a trip to San Diego, and I was feeling some back pain when we returned. It was so painful that I considered calling a physical therapist, and I was taking pain relievers. I was able to go to work, but I had twingy feelings in my back. Then, about three weeks after this new sensation began, I was alone with the kids one afternoon. In an effort to calm my daughter, I tried to pick her up when she firmly resisted. I could feel my back strain, but at the time I had no pain.

In the back of my mind, I was very concerned.

I never got better, I got worse. I've never been back to work.

The worst part of this injury is that I cannot sit. If I could be in a wheelchair, I could get wheeled around and go places. I could use a motorized cart. I could go in the car. I could go places. It's very hard to do anything when you can't sit.

It took five months before a back specialist made the diagnosis of internal disk disruption. And, because two disks were involved, there was little likelihood of help from surgery.

The recommendation we decided to try was to simulate the surgery situation, which was to immobilize my spine by fusion. The surgeon recommended a body cast. I agreed to this.

The cast went from above my breast all the way down to mid thigh, immobilizing the hip joint completely. It turned out to be very traumatic. I couldn't keep up with my personal hygiene. No one had prepared me for what accessories would be required with the body cast.

We went ahead in July 1994, for surgery. Anterior fusion under laperoscopy surgery—quite revolutionary for back surgery. The doctors implanted titanium cages filled with bone grafts from my hip. The titanium was to give it support and structure, and the bone grafts were to grow and eventually fuse my back. Fusion would diminish the movement of my spine and reduce the back pain. It was supposed to be one surgery with a week's hospital stay. I ended up in the hospital for twenty-two days with all sorts of medical complications.

I had arrived home on a Monday evening and by Thursday afternoon I started to have severe pins and needles in both feet. I could barely walk. As a result of this, my doctor enforced bed rest.

I began to feel fear for the first time. I "hit the wall" when I realized I might not get better according to my doctor's timetable. Here we are, thinking about vacations we've already missed from the year before, our child-care expenses, the quality of our family life, and although the doctor never said I might not walk again, it actually hit me that I might not.

My husband, John, had been holding the fort for more than a year, and here I was back to square one. The future looked grimly overwhelming. He expressed himself as a single parent. He started getting more testy. He would say things like, "You have GOT to get better. I can't keep up, doing all of this." I understand his rage. He had been functioning as a superdad and a very supportive husband while being a doctor on the side. And all I was doing was lying helpless in our bed.

Over time, I developed benign vertigo because of the immobilization. Months would go by when I would get up and the room would spin around. I was told that this happens from not exercising and being in one position for too long. My heart rate also went up; normally my pulse is between sixty-five and eighty doing normal activity. My doctor said I had astronaut syndrome, because I was always lying down without any exertional stress on my body.

In April 1995 I had another surgery. It went well. By the time I had left the hospital, I was up for half-hour stretches and walking up and down stairs. I didn't have a twinge in my body. I felt great!

Upon returning home, I felt the urge simply to cut back the pain medicine since I didn't have pain. Suddenly, I had pain again. Emotionally, this was the hardest time. I bottomed out. I was so close to a great recovery and then the pain returned.

In July, we found a physical therapist who worked on my

shoulders. In addition, I hired a Feldenkrais therapist who came twice a week. With physical therapy three times a week, I felt I was doing something to make me feel better and tone me up. The hands on my body made me feel so much better.

The physical therapy in conjunction with the pain program (medication) has been the key to my recovery. It is the only way that I can get out of bed for a little while and work toward healing.

I spend much of my time in bed thinking about how to improve my general health and fitness. Because of the inactivity of bed rest, I've tried to eat more sensibly. I eat a lot of fruit and veggies. I've gotten away from sweets and turned to fruits. When you don't exercise, your cholesterol goes up. I've changed all of my eating habits.

I am up and about for an hour a day. I'm very involved, and I feel that our family life has improved. I've learned to be assertive about not missing family events or milestones. We traded in the two cars we had and bought a van so that I could be laid out in the back of it when I need to be transported. It makes everyone happy when I can go along to an event, even though wherever we land, I am transported straight to the massage table.

There have been and continue to be many positive aspects of having been bedridden and being home all the time. Although I miss practicing medicine terribly, I love running the household from my bed. The kids have helped to make this manageable and enjoyable. When it's time for piano lessons, they answer the door and set themselves up. They know I am listening from my upstairs bed. At night, I time them while they practice. Before each piece, they yell up the stairs to tell me the names of the songs.

I coordinate all of the kids' outings by telephone and make sure their homework is done. We do clothes and toy shopping together by catalog, which has become quite a fun process. I take pride in how they look and they have learned a sense of style earlier than many children their age.

My new approach is based on a major switch in my attitude. You can either sink or swim in a situation like this. I've made the choice to accept my situation and come to terms with a completely new identity. I used to feel very sorry for myself and isolated. With acceptance, I'm not only getting better, but I'm more integrated into our family life. I'm the mom who's always around, and I'm growing to love it. My husband really appreciates my positive attitude and is relieved of worrying so much about me and all the details of each of our children's welfare.

I enjoy being the family command post. All phone calls come through me. The neighborhood, soccer leagues, and school community know me as "The Timekeeper" for everyone's schedules. I also have better friendships with the children's friends and their parents. This has been really fun.

Being on bed rest has given me the gift of having a much more intimate relationship with the children. They feel how receptive I am to them, and they know I am always available if they need anything.

I wouldn't have made it this far without a few key discoveries that everyone on bed rest should know about. Wearing a watch and labeling your medicine so you can see it easily (side and top of vial) have reduced the hassle factor of my pain program. The wedge pillow has been my greatest source of physical comfort. My "Grab It Stick" can pick up paper, pencils, and very small things. It's the best! They come in all sorts of colors, which is fun!

The portable phone has reduced neck aches and worrying about knocking anything off the side table. Remote control is essential for enjoying TV and feeling independent. Cable TV has added to my appreciation of television as it has been very educational and entertaining.

The items I have used on bed rest that have helped me the most are as follows:

❏ Beeper for my husband
❏ Walker
❏ Massage table—for the outings that you can't miss
❏ Commode—portable nonflush toilet if bathroom is too far from your room
❏ Back brace

- ❏ Washcloth for hands and face
- ❏ Straws
- ❏ Mug with family photo
- ❏ Personal needs table: creams, medicine, drinks, note cards, tissue
- ❏ Your own set of house keys to drop out of window down to someone in the case of an emergency
- ❏ Makeup with mirror—I've had fun with this for myself and with my daughter
- ❏ Electric toothbrush (eliminates the arm motion/body motion)
- ❏ Small pet—fish, cat, hamster

Madeleine (54 years old)

My medical problem was environmental illness, from which I suffered severely for twelve years. This illness is autoimmune; my immune system was compromised. I was often tired. I "got sick" easily. I had to spend long periods of time in bed resting to prevent myself from getting sick or recuperating from an illness like a cold or flu. I live in northern California. I reacted to the dampness and the mold in winter, to the air pollution in the summer, and to the pollen in the spring and fall.

My illness really frightened me. I would be so sick at times that I had to stay in bed for days, a week, or more. I never knew how long I would have to be in bed, when the illness would end, or whether I would recover from each bout of the illness. Sometimes I could barely digest my food. At other times my body ached all over. I had severe respiratory problems like bronchitis. I would also be weakened by kidney-bladder infections. These are all typical illnesses associated with the syndrome called environmental illness.

In the early years, I was consumed with fear that I would never be able to get out of bed or that I would never want to get out of bed. I was afraid I wouldn't survive. One bright sunny day, I couldn't stand to stay in bed any longer. I had the emotional energy I needed to get up and go outside, even though I could barely walk from weakness and fatigue. My partner drove me to the Berkeley Marina, where I found a large, beautiful, grassy area. I lay on the grass and felt its richness and softness. I felt warmed and vitalized by the bright sun. I marveled at how much I was enjoying this experience. Rather than just resting in bed, I could rest in a beautiful, lush, sunny meadow! I had found a way to enjoy myself even though I was so sick! For this reason, I knew I could and would survive.

I began to think of the large grassy area whenever I had to rest in bed. Using this association, I realized the possibility of enjoying my time resting. I was freed from others' expectations, from needing to please others. I felt healthier in bed because my limits were clearer, as were the limits of what I could do. I felt freed from having to do so much all the time. I couldn't do very much. I was too sick. All that I could do besides resting in bed was work and take care of my basic survival needs. Bed rest had freed me from the demands of the outside world.

I functioned very well as a therapist during this phase of my illness. I saw clients in a clean room in my home, where I did not have the distractions of my bedroom. My experience on bed rest helped me develop a new level of awareness and openness to my own bodily and emotional processes. With my clients, I was centered, sensitive, and open. Focusing so much of my energy on my own healing helped me support and be sensitive to my clients' needs for healing. I was more present with my clients than when I was higher functioning, i.e. busily fulfilling what I perceived as the demands of external reality.

I learned to enjoy just being. I found meaning in my existence from "being" rather than doing or achieving. It was OK to rest and watch old movies on TV. Thanks to my illness, I felt permission for the first time to enjoy resting in bed. Now that I am healthy again, I still try to give myself that permission—to enjoy just being. I try not to do too many things, and if I am tired, I rest. I don't push myself like I used to. If I don't get something done, it doesn't get done. I have a new perspective on living. I am living more for me, rather than for other people. I like my work and I work hard. Then, I rest. I accept that I don't have to work all the time. I have learned, thanks to the bed rest of my illness, how to rest. And how to enjoy resting.

Owen (51 years old)

Ever since the early sixties, when I first discovered serious cycling, I had dreamed, like a devout Moslem, of going on haj to Mecca, of making a pilgrimage to Europe. This was the world epicenter of the sport, the place with the most races, the highest standards, and the greatest public standards.

Unfortunately, a season in Europe was no idle financial enterprise. It took me a half dozen years of savings before I was able finally to make the plunge. That was in 1972, at the relatively advanced age of twenty-six.

I joined three other Americans in a flat near Grenoble, France. I bought a used car and a bike and we were soon into the swing of the bike life. It was the dream life: eat, sleep, and ride. Like monks in the nearby monastery of the Grand Chartreuse we lived a focused life. That life demanded a balance of effort with recovery. Sometimes that balance wasn't maintained. We often left at dawn to drive to a race, frequently racing in freezing rain and even snow (it was the coldest summer of the century). We'd return at night to a cold dinner and colder shower.

These and other stresses notwithstanding, I felt fit and ready for any adversity. One night in late June we rode a nighttime criterium under the street lights of Chambery. As usual the rain was lashing down, but by now we were inured to its effects.

Inevitably, someone had a lapse of attention, his bike slid out from under him, and it was my misfortune to be directly behind. I hit the downed rider in his back and was catapulted through the air onto my back with a resounding whack. It was at this point, my focus abruptly shifted from the idealized cycling life to hell in bed.

Once I was cleared from the course and my buddies found me shivering on the sidelines, they did their merciful best to get me back to the apartment and into my bed. They laid me out, wished me well, and rushed off to eat, clean up, and get ready for the next day's outing. The ensuing quiet let me take stock of things.

The pain was located in my lower back just left of center. My father had complained of similar pains, something about his sacroiliac, and I wondered if there was a relationship. If so, then I knew nothing was broken, that somehow a nerve was pinched. This self-diagnosis was only a minor relief because the pain was, in my experience, beyond description.

I wanted to take some of my clothes off and crawl under the covers. The least movement ignited shocks. In two hours I finally got my jacket off; I gave up on the rest. By grabbing the blanket, rolling one way and then back across them, I was finally able to get between the sheets.

If I lay in certain positions and didn't move, the pain was bearable and for the first time I was able to relax a bit. The pool of sweat I lay in began to dry up.

However, the tenuous balance began to be undermined by the increasing urge to pee. Jesus, what to do? NO way could I get out of bed, let alone navigate to the bathroom. Then I spied my water glass. Oh sweet salvation! I threw what little was left out the open window next to the bed and then filled the glass almost to the top. This, too, went out the window and down eight stories. I hoped no one below was leaning out and wondering where this urine downpour was coming from.

I had never felt so bewildered or trapped. If I lay just right, the pain was more threatening than actual. I could do absolutely nothing.

Boring? You bet! The hours dragged by. Sometime after dark the guys returned. They were good enough to sit around for a while, give me a description of the race results and their day's adventures, get me some food, and carry me to the bathroom. They got my water bottle off my bike so I could have my own water supply. They also piled a stack of French bike magazines next to me, the only reading matter in the house.

They were as solicitous as they could be, but I knew they

were in France for the same reason I was, to grab the chance of a lifetime. In short, I was mostly on my own. Beyond the fact that I couldn't join them, my situation made them uncomfortable. They soon resumed eating in the kitchen.

The constant low-grade pain that could erupt at the slightest wrong move was a perpetual aggravation. But I was used to this type of adversity. Every bikie is. How to suffer is cycling's first lesson. But there is suffering and there is suffering, and the boredom soon came to weigh on me far more than the pain. My French was still rudimentary, so the magazines were mostly valuable for the pictures. I had language books and studied them several times a day and went to great lengths to decipher passages in the magazines, but I longed for some easy entertaining reading. Occasionally one of the guys would get me a *Time* magazine or *Herald Tribune*, but the tourist areas where such fare was offered were usually far from the sites of bike races.

There was no one to phone. Not only did I not really know anyone in town, there were no phones. You went to the post office for that. No TV. Endless gray skies.

I was familiar with the Zen idea of thinking of nothing, sort of trying not to try. I remembered a psychology article I'd read some time back about the benefits of going mad. At the time the reality necessary for that was so far from my own I'd only dimly grasped the article's meaning, but now it was making more sense every day. If you could, in your mind, make a complete break with the world and enter a nicer space of your own creation, a whole order of difficulty could be resolved. I wasn't quite ready for that yet, but contemplating its attractive possibilities was now no longer a vision dimly perceived; now it was a potential solution lurking on the other side of a nearby wall.

Beyond boredom and pain was frustration. I was perfectly familiar with Victor Frankl's admonition in his famous book, *Man's Search for Meaning,* that our ultimate freedom lies in our ability to choose our attitude toward any situation. I played with the idea a lot. (God knows, I had the time!) I tried it out in my head. Now I could really learn French. Now I could really discover myself through meditation. Now I could put cycling into its proper role as only a part of life. It actually helped me get through the days.

Thank God for the view from the room. Meditating on the interplay of mountains and weather provided not only the form of sweet entertainment but also the only peace I found.

After three weeks I got a surprise visit from the uncle of a French bikie who knew there had been four of us Americans and had inquired as to why there were now only three. When told, the old man came by and pushed and prodded my back and slapped on a heat plaster laced with "phenalgon," a cream derived from an extract of marmot liver and so hot that if you rubbed yourself all over, you could, I'm sure, run naked in the arctic with impunity.

Whatever he did, it changed something, and the next day I took my first halting steps to the bathroom. In two more days I went outside and in a week I was able to get back on the salvation machine, my bike, although it was another month before I got back to the races. I was stronger mentally than ever. I had just proven to myself that I had depths I didn't know I had. I had just spent the heart of the summer discovering a new form of long mountain climbing. It sure felt good to transfer the iron will back to the bike.

Susan (39 years old)

My bed rest experience occurred in the heart of winter. Frequent snow cover added a silence and stillness that conveniently supported my situation. The weather and time of year helped me relax into a cocoon of calm. My initial reaction to being put on bed rest for preterm labor was outrage. It was a shock to my system to be forced into bed rest. I had planned, after all, to be one of those who exercised right through my pregnancy. I had been accustomed to running, aerobics, etc. I worked in an art studio and was on my feet all day, doing art.

Now, I couldn't even walk to the toilet without fear of contractions which could, at any point, send me back to the hospital.

I had been hospitalized seven times prior to this for preterm labor symptoms.

During my first hospitalization, my husband left for a three-week business trip. I was already angry, and, on top of it I now felt very abandoned. I had terrible times of fear. My mother came to stay with me. She made me feel so loved and protected with her care and support. When my husband returned from his business trip, and for the remainder of the pregnancy, he was available and supportive of me in every way. No other visitors came, but a couple of friends stayed in touch by phone.

My husband's good care is what made me feel most comfortable settling into bed rest. He took care of cooking, cleaning, shopping, and everything! Small but loving gestures such as drawing a bath, fluffing pillows, massaging my shoulders, and frequent kisses helped so much! I also relied on other, less personalized things such as Tylenol, antacids, heating pad, and Tiger Balm. Since I had been hospitalized several times, I learned to pack quickly, never forgetting these items and my pillow. These items can be difficult or impossible to get in a hospital.

I tried to keep a daily schedule, especially while I was home bedridden. It included morning papers, lunch, a nap, one soap opera, more reading, music, and dinner. Once I settled calmly into acceptance, bed rest was more peaceful. I also read a series of novels by Tony Hillerman. For me it was the right combination of suspense—to hold my interest—and "poetry" from the Native American aspect. I would highly recommend them.

I ate only for nutrition. I was not hungry because of the medication. I could only eat small quantities, as I could not sit up to aid digestion. It was too painful to sit. I ate soup and salad, yogurt and fruit. (What a difference in my second pregnancy that did not involve bed rest . . . pizza, chocolate, and all!).

I moved very little. I was too afraid to do anything that might cause a miscarriage. I probably should have had massage or something. I was a twisted pretzel after months of bed rest. My most physical act was when my husband and I cuddled. We were afraid to do too much! My husband did receive sexual caressing from me. For the most part, we were in another "space" in our relationship and existence. Sex wasn't very important at this time in our lives. The fetus was in danger, we had to tread lightly.

I was very lucky to have two important people in my life respond in such a supportive way. They helped nurture my courage and faith to carry on. My belief in God was also a tremendous benefit.

Phyllis (57 years old)

I woke up one morning in November literally unable to walk. I was terrified that something was wrong with my hip replacement. My surgeon x-rayed my hip and determined I had a complication with sciatica and would have to lie on my back. Ice and rest would cure me.

Fortunately, I have a cottage industry. I design and hand-sew silk flowers. The Christmas season is my busiest time, and I had to continue to manufacture my product. So, I lay on my back and sewed away. With CDs playing to keep me company, I made all the flowers I needed to fill my orders, kept my sanity, and healed my problem. I read a great deal. At one point I had my husband gather all of my large art books. On a makeshift table next to my bed, I gave myself a comprehensive art history course! When it was time to begin walking and exercising my hip and back, I wasn't finished with my coursework. I carved out some time during each day to fulfill what became a passionate curiosity and personal side interest.

My time in bed gave me an opening to a facet of life I would never have had the time to appreciate or explore to the degree and pleasure that I did.

Jennifer (37 years old)

I've always fantasized about pregnancy and motherhood. I always envisioned myself active and definitely processing that commonly talked about "glow." I did not picture the experience

I had. My child was born prematurely—that he was born at all seems miraculous to me. My OB-Gyn told me, shortly after the birth of my son, that my pregnancy was the second worst she'd seen in all her years of practice. I salute the woman who's in first place and all those women I met in the hospital while our babies were ripening on the vine, next to the lines of IV poles, bedpans, nightmare medications . . . and clocks that seemed to have stopped.

I have always felt that when I fear something, the fear will lessen if I know more about the thing I'm fearing. Each doctor I saw (and I saw a different one every day of the week) had a different idea about what was going on and what they were going to do. The more I tried to find out, the more confused I became. I had such a feeling of helplessness.

Initially I'd been sentenced to my home—the couch or the bed for the duration of my pregnancy. I was allowed to get up to use the bathroom and fix a light lunch. The isolation in itself was a challenge.

I remember bumping into a friend in a store two days after I was put on bed rest. She wanted to know what I was doing out of bed. I realized right then it hadn't quite sunk in. I had to stop doing everything, no more just one more errand. I had to stop. It was Christmastime. I have to say I was excited about the time of year, the anticipation of a baby, and the buzz in the air. All of this kept me going during this first phase of bed rest. Then it turned really cold and gray. Depression set in. My husband is a packrat and every day I watched my house go to hell a little further. I couldn't get up to do the things I wanted to. There was junk mail everywhere, newspapers, dirty dishes. Laundry I had started right as I was put on bed rest stayed out in a basket for the entire time of my "imprisonment." I felt alone and help-less, and that made me even more depressed.

The hospital bed rest started without any planning and not much warning. A one-day trip to be monitored for contractions led into a night-long bout. I received countless shots of terbutaline and never left the hospital again for two and a half months. When my son was born, he had to stay in the hospital for two more months. Our whole hospital experience was almost five months long. I knew the security guards, janitors, and kitchen help all by first name.

The time in the hospital was one of the most psychologially and physically rigorous I've ever experienced. I was monitored for contractions around the clock. The large white belt that was constantly wrapped around my belly felt like the most uncomfortable daily uniform. There was a constant sound of paper tape flowing from the monitor attached to my body. I spent hours staring at the monitor, a tall glass of water, and the ever-familiar straw. Sometimes it felt like it took me all day to get that straw into my mouth and sip. The medication I was on was hellish. the combination of terbutaline and magnesium sulfide is what did me in. Mag sulfide is a muscle relaxer. The nurses maxed me out on it. I couldn't move my body, but my mind was racing in a torturous state of anxiety. The goal was to get my contractions to stop and not go into "real labor" and deliver the baby too soon.

One night, I was told it looked as if I was going to lose the baby. They almost called my husband. A nurse was trying to teach me some relaxation techniques, and she asked if she could give me a massage. I'd never had one before. She stayed with me for a couple of hours, calming me and dragging every ounce of tension from my body with her incredibly strong and healing hands. This saved my sanity and, I believe, the life of my baby.

When the contractions were finally under control, I graduated to the high-risk wing of the hospital. It was nice to see some light and life and a change. I usually don't like change, but this change came close to being a religious experience for me. Initially, I wanted a room to myself, but looking back, I think it was helpful to share a room. At least something happened to distract me from time to time. I learned more about problem pregnancies than I ever dreamed of. I also met people I'm sure I would never have met otherwise. Some are now very close friends.

The whole experience felt like a crash course in crisis management. What usually worked for me in the past didn't work under these circumstances. I've had years of therapy because of anxiety/depression and panic disorder . . . I though I'd trained myself fairly well. I found myself desperate to get a handle on something that would really help me cope.

The strength to carry on came from supportive people. I suggest if you are on bed rest, for any reason, designate helpers. You will need this. I would have surely died if there had been no one. If you define a job for someone to do, whether you're paying them or not, you have an agreement. I don't have to feel guilty or uncomfortable asking for that job to be done. People all around us possess incredible healing powers just by being who they are. It doesn't take but a minute to keep someone going for a week. Friends and family can do so much to help. They need you to tell them what you want.

There were times when I didn't want to see anyone, or so I thought. I got quite proficient at speaking up for myself. It's amazing how we think we don't want to see a soul and then suddenly we are weeping in gratitude for the kindness and healing that comes with a visit. I did this a lot. I loved contact with people. It was helpful to have people affirm that this was truly a difficult experience. My husband's aunt called me every night like clockwork. She only talked for a short while, but having that consistency was wonderful. It also helped to have people listen when I needed to talk or vent. A hug when I broke into tears helped recharge me. It also helped to hear what other people were doing. Real-life stories gave me life and hope. I would visualize life beyond where I lay.

Besides people, there were things that helped me cope. The one on the top of the list was my Walkman. Music—blessed music—and a self-hypnosis tape got me through. The tape helped me go to sleep like nothing else could. I finally got to the point where I could calm down and fall asleep just by closing my eyes and imagining putting the tape on, starting the breathing, and bingo . . . I'd be out in five minutes. At first, it would take at least an hour if it worked at all. I still use the techniques if I ever really need them.

Realizing that the Walkman made a huge difference for me, I became somewhat obsessed about having a good supply of batteries. I would burn through them. I have a wonderful friend who didn't laugh or tease me when I told him I lived in fear that I'd run out of batteries in the middle of the night. He made a trip to Costco and brought me an enormous supply. This has made many memories for me over the years when I reach for "another battery."

Flowers helped a lot. Anything living uplifted my spirits! One day a friend brought in some freshly picked rosemary. That night when I couldn't get to sleep, I reached for the rosemary and began breathing in its fragrance. Hospitals have a definite "smell." The bedridden body and soul need sources of life! Every once in a while a friend would get permission to wheel my bed outside on the patio. This was totally therapeutic. The sun recharged me so completely . . . I wished we could all have our hospital beds outside. I think people in similar situations would heal a lot faster.

One day, one of the nurses brought in needlework and watercolors. I never watched TV, and I rarely got beyond the first page of the many books people brought me. However, I was surprised by the amount of pleasure I received from the needlework and watercolors. I never would have guessed this would be so calming and fulfilling.

I found comfort in having familiar things from home close to me: a picture of my dog, my pillow, my cross, some favorite foods not on the hospital menu, a candle, a stuffed bear that I clung to in front of everyone! Integrating this into my bedside existence made me feel safe and comfortable.

I was home for only two days (after two and a half months in the hospital), when I returned to the hospital for an emergency C-section. I now have a beautiful, delightful, healthy seven-year-old boy! If someone were to tell me I'd have to do it all again in order to keep him, I'd do it immediately with no regrets! He is the biggest blessing of my life.

Perrin (36 years old)

It was a hot Labor Day weekend, I was 26 weeks pregnant with my third child when I began bleeding. When I called my doctor, he wasn't sure what was occurring but it was thought that there may be a tear or hole in the placenta which might have occurred during the amniocentesis. Nothing would be known for sure until delivery.

When we arrived at the hospital and were told I would return home in ten weeks or as soon as the baby arrived, we both went into shock! My husband was numb! However, with two small children running around, there wasn't time for delay. I jumped into practical mode immediately.

I have had four pregnancies prior to this. The first two ended in miscarriages at three months. The second two are my beautiful sons, who at the time of this pregnancy were two and a half and five.

I called an old friend/day-care giver who generously agreed to take over the first week. Each day, my husband dropped off my younger son at Leslie's home and then delivered the older boy to school. When kindergarten was over, friends dropped him off to join his brother. My husband picked them up each evening. Leslie was a lifesaver! After one week, my mother arrived from California to stay for three weeks. The plan was that she would stay until the baby arrived. My mother-in-law would arrive during the fourth week.

It took a week before my husband began to talk again and react to life! I think he and the boys missed me very much, especially because it all happened so suddenly. My kindergartner had just started school. He was overwhelmed with no mom at home and a new school. I felt very guilty that I couldn't be there for him.

Once my mother arrived, home life settled down and the boys were in their familiar schedule. Soon, conflicts arose between Grandma's and my parenting style. I heard a lot about this from daily visits, from both the kids and grandmother! I felt helpless and yet extremely grateful that the basics were very well taken care of. I accepted that life wouldn't be ideal for anyone, but it could be very good given the circumstances.

My local support system was beyond anything I would have ever expected. My friends and neighbors sent meals to the house. They organized car pools for the kids. One family even traded cars so the grandmothers could drive (automatic)! Other friends contacted volunteer organizations that helped with deliveries. Books arrived weekly.

Our relatives were loving and extremely attentive. Each of our mothers dropped everything to travel from out of state to be grandmothers in action! Other family members called me at the hospital regularly. I actually began to feel like a Queen for a Day.

I spent much of my time reading, enjoying the newspaper, and watching the news. These kinds of activities were refreshing given the number of distractions that regularly occurred at home. I worked on and finished a cross stitch pillow for the baby. My involvement with a volunteer organization continued. I held meetings and presented slide shows in my room for the organization. I tried really hard to keep my own normal routine without giving up on planned events—just moved place and time!

The food in the hospital was acceptable, but without some of my favorite treats sent in, I would have gone crazy. Pizza was delivered whenever the family came for dinner. Also, chocolates were sent to me, which I hid from the doctors!

The hospital staff was fantastic. I really enjoyed getting to know the nurses. They seemed to read my mind whenever I had a specific worry. For instance, I was concerned with my muscles losing strength. A physical therapist arrived just in time to show me some upper body exercises with an elastic band. The nurses provided body massages! I missed being physical, and I missed being out of doors. We were having the most beautiful fall I could remember (I could see a little from my window). Being wheeled out on weekends by my family cheered me a great deal. A couple of times they wheeled me to a park near the hospital.

I missed the physical intimacy I enjoy with my husband. "Making love" in the hospital consisted of late-night visits without the children, lying on the bed together, snuggling, talking, and watching TV. My husband usually fell asleep; he was exhausted with kids, work, grandmothers, and visits back and forth. I knew he loved me.

Many times in the hospital, I felt like a prisoner who had to greet everyone who dropped in. Sometimes I took the phone off the hook so I could rest. I was surprised by some visits from people I hardly knew while others, like a neighbor across the street whose children were our children's playmates, never came. I found out later that she hates hospitals and lost her first husband in one. Most of all, I depended on daily visits from my husband and the kids. I was very disappointed if they didn't make it. They were my life and link to normalcy. Many times I felt isolated, helpless, guilty. Many times people would tell me, "take advantage of this—you'll never have this free time again!" Wheelchair visits to the nursery and staff neonatologist helped me to realize I was doing the smart thing by being in the hospital for immediate assistance. The possibility of hemorrhaging was high, and it was foolish to risk the baby's or my life.

I made the right decision. I delivered a daughter, Abby, two pounds, nine ounces at 31 ½ weeks. She was breathing on her own, and after fifty days came home from the ICU. Everyone is healthy and happy. It was all worth it!

Ross (35 years old)

In the spring of 1992, while traveling, I became sick with a viral illness. I expected that it would pass within a couple of weeks, but it lingered for the duration of my trip. When I returned home I no longer had the signs of acute infection in my throat, lungs, and sinuses, but other disturbing and frightening symptoms were developing. The fatigue I experienced was now so severe that not only was I confined to lying in bed, but just to breathe seemed a great effort. Every cell in my body felt as if it were burning with pain. Sleep was frequently disturbed and seemed to offer no relief and no sense of replenishment. It was a journey into a hell of physical pain and mental and emotional anguish.

After a thorough physical exam and testing, the doctors I saw said they could not find anything to explain these disabling, painful, and frightening symptoms. Eventually, I would receive a diagnosis of chronic fatigue syndrome, but at the outset no one I saw could explain what was happening. I desperately wished for some diagnosis, something that was known and could be cured. I was hoping for some way out of this experience of hell.

After two weeks passed in what seemed like unbearable torture and despair, I found the way out of this nightmare. Not through any form of dissociation or pain control, but in the simplest secret of surrender and self-recognition.

Ten years previous to the onset of my illness, my father's death at the young age of forty-six, confronted me with the fact that this life in a physical body was impermanent and could be taken away at any moment. Although his death was a shock and a great loss, it sparked something inside: a longing to know, "What is permanent?" "Is there something deeper than this apparent life?"

After months and years of soul-searching, meditating, and experiencing various levels of self and being, meeting new friends and teachers, I traveled in the fall of 1991, to India. It was there that I met Gangaji. In meeting her, my search for that everlasting peace I had had glimpses of after my father had died ended. In the lineage of Ramana Maharshi, a renowned sage who lived in India in the first part of this century, Gangaji's teaching was a direct, living transmission of silence. "Be still and realize that you are That which you are seeking." Her message was so simple and clear. Her presence and her words stopped the momentum of my perpetual mental activity. My attention was redirected. "Who am I?" "Who is this one who is seeking?"

Through this meeting, and my willingness to be still and make this inquiry, the deepest secret of my being was revealed. What was revealed is That which cannot be known, but That Which I AM.

It was made clear to me through this revelation that my true nature is not an experience, but That in which all experiences come and go. Wonderful experiences didn't need to be held on to, and horrific experiences didn't need to be avoided. Regardless of outer circumstances, regardless of states of body, mind, or emotion—one's attention can be at rest in the truth of who one is.

I was instructed to experience fully and directly everything that appeared in consciousness, with the understanding that no experience is needed for this revelation of being. In staying true to what was revealed as the truth of my Self, life would unfold in bliss and gratitude. In turning away from the truth by reidentifying as a "somebody" rather than the Source and essence of all bodies, one would again experience suffering. I awoke at this time to the realization that I would be tested in many ways. I was soon to find this out, through this experience of an unexplained, painful, and disabling illness.

After two weeks of the worst misery I have ever known, I woke up to the fact that I was suffering deeply, and that I knew from my learning that suffering was caused by misidentification—not by circumstances. I was suffering because I again identified with being my body. I deeply wanted to avoid this unpleasant and terrifying experience, and I deeply desired a happy ending to this chapter of crisis.

Once I acknowledged the truth about why I was suffering, I became aware that my deepest commitment and longing was to realize directly the truth of who I am in every moment and in whatever circumstances appear. I surrendered resistance and opened my heart to the experience I was given. I stopped wanting it to be different.

For better or for worse, I was there. I knew that however unpleasant this experience was and may continue to be, that it was a great opportunity for deeper revelation of being.

I continued to surrender to the outcome of what would unfold with my body's health. My attention stopped spinning in the hellish realm of hope and despair. In this surrender, deep and sweet peace revealed itself. The pain was still present. The severe fatigue was still present. The sleepless nights still happened.

Yet the experience was no longer a hell. Everything that was happening with my body was now held in a realization of being That which is limitless, conscious, love itself. It was now obvious and clear that nothing needed to happen, and nothing needed to be avoided. I could let go completely and be at peace with whatever may unfold in the appearance of this life. No words can describe the peace and fulfillment of this realization.

Almost five years have passed since the onset of my experience of bed rest. I continue to experience disabling fatigue and pain, and I continue to experiment with a variety of treatments to regain health. I have made some improvement, and my intuition tells me that in time I will regain my health. I have periods where my body seems to be doing well, only to relapse again. These relapses have been very painful and disappointing. And yet, the disappointment passes quickly because it continues to be obvious that what I really want, what I really love and who I really am are all the same. All is Love. And this is always available to be freshly realized regardless of circumstances.

There have been many challenges during this time, and yet these years have been the richest and most joyful I have ever known. I consider myself to be the luckiest man in the world. Everything I was previously wanting in the outside world has found its fulfillment in the deepening realization of the truth of That Which I AM. Not separate from anything. In spite of my physical limitations, many aspects of my life in which I previously struggled, are now flowering effortlessly.

This time on bed rest has been so precious. The time to be still is such a gift. No effort, knowledge, or training is required to discover what I am speaking of. It is simply recognizing who you really are, always have been, and always will be. What is required is a willingness to stop everything, and be still—for at least a single moment. In this moment the mind is directed to discover its source. Find out directly, "Who am I?" Whatever your circumstances may be, "Who is it that is aware of all of this?"

If you find that this is your time for bed rest, then you have been given a precious opportunity. You can find out who you are: deeper than any thought, any sensation, any feeling.

In my experience, there is nothing more important than this inquiry. All of our conditioning tells us that we should be "doing" something, and that just being silent and still is a waste of time. But all that can be done, and all that can be known will in time be washed away like sand castles on the beach. There is That which cannot be washed away, and You Are That.

I wish you good luck.

Joel (48 years old)

Joel is a screenplay writer and artist. At the time of his back injury, he was Francis Ford Coppola's personal aide. His story was sent to me in the following screenplay form:

FADE IN

INTERIORS—BEAKINS STORAGE—DAY

Our hero, Joel Adelman, is schlepping boxes of sound-track tape for Francis Coppola and Zoetrope Studios (the envy and wonder of the civilized world, home of proven hits).

He seems a lost soul, consigned to an existential hell of endless, dimly lit wooden corridors. Using his best straight-back, tight-gut, bent-knee technique, he lifts a fatal box of sound-effects reels (*Dragon Slayer:* Dragon's footsteps through mud, water, across stone surfaces). Joel's expression (and life for years to come) changes as he feels his lower back muscles give way with a sound effect, for an audience of one, like a sheet of thick plastic tearing.

CUT TO ONE YEAR LATER

INTERIORS—JOEL'S BEDROOM, ST. HELENA, CALIFORNIA—DAY

Lucky for Joel, he's married to a loving sweetie and has a thirteen-year-old daughter, because at this point there's not much he can do for himself. He spends his time trying not to move, cough, or even breathe too hard because all of that sends his lower back into spasms—thirty-second torture zones where he is transfixed by an invisible railroad spike rammed right into L5S1. Lying on one's back hour after hour, one's lungs fill with fluid, and eventually one is forced to cough and suffer the consequences.

Part of his depression is that although he is thirty-one, Joel feels about a hundred years old. He looks very defeated. The ten-foot walk to the bathroom is a great big deal. He cannot find comfort anywhere, even his underwear is a struggle as it is not designed for his blown disks. Nor are his shoes and socks. He can't walk or drive anywhere. All of his musculature is slowly melting away. Joel looks frustrated and angry.

Three doctors have recommended surgery—"We can get you on the table next Tuesday." But Joel, your humble narrator, has the sneaking suspicion he can beat the rap without getting sliced and diced.

JOEL SPEAKING:
I have never had a seriously debilitating illness or injury before. My initial reaction was shock and outrage. My body, which still seemed 99 percent perfectly healthy, was rendered inert due to the 1 percent that had muntinied. I was furious. I was also afraid. How bad was this going to get? Would I recover function and to what degree? During the first couple of months I was getting an education on what had actually occurred, what the various treatments were, what was the likely outcome of each treatment, recovery time, etc. At some point during this process, I simply decided I would get better without surgery, either on my own or with the help of body workers. The various orthopedists dismissed this option. Today, I am glad I am stubborn and determined.

My situation would have been very difficult without my family around to help. Just their presence and concern made me feel more courageous and hopeful, even after two years of pain and disability. Oddly enough, the fact that my wife and daughter made constant fun of me, my crab walk, the amount of time it took to do anything, etc., helped me a lot! Being able to see the comic and absurd side of the situation kept me from taking myself too seriously.

One night I was alone in the house, Manuela and Mia had gone out shopping. I was lying on my back in bed, knees up on two pillows. It was winter, and I was wearing a warm sweater. Manuela had turned on the heat before she left and now the sweater was too hot. I carefully and slowly tried to sneak the sweater off without my back knowing. An hour later, after numerous spasms, I was totally worn out. I had only been able to maneuver my sweater over my head, so now my head was stuck in the sweater. I burst into tears of rage and frustration, and that's how my family found me, crying with my head in the sweater.

Pain is physically and spiritually exhausting. It is draining, and yet, like many other people, I came to the conclusion that I'd rather be in pain than feel as numb, dumb, and dead as the painkillers and anti-inflammatories made me feel. Every now and then, some relief is welcome, but for me, medication is a downward spiral when relied on every day.

I took every advantage of the contrasting energies welling up within me. I channeled my anger and feistiness toward healing. I used this powerful energy to be strong and willful against an enemy that at times felt simply too big to fight. I used my quieter energy for healing meditation and visualization. While in surrender mode, I actually felt better. The peacefulness of acceptance calmed my otherwise strong male tendencies to fight. In combination, these energies supported an inner faith I had in the healing powers of my own body and my own life force. With this, in addition to the love and support of my family, I began to move beyond the pain and disability.

Martha (47 years old)

At the time I was bedridden, I was working twenty hours per week. My employer was very supportive of my triplet pregnancy. He let me use sick leave and maternity leave.

My husband worked long hours, but when he was home, he was very attentive. It also helped that his parents visited twice a week and brought dinner. Three other men who were students at the local university shared our house and were pleasant but not too involved. We hired a live-in cook, a student who made my meals and everyone's dinner.

My favorite meal was fresh-squeezed orange juice with Metamucil for breakfast. I usually ate a snack of apples and cheese, a sandwich for lunch, and a normal dinner with everyone. Every day, I had four meat and dairy servings, lots of fruit—nothing fried, spicy, or sweet. I was a happy beached whale.

I had little trouble tolerating bed rest. Once my coffee table was converted to a little trolley, I was able to reach the things I needed: my gallon jug of water, my books, my lunch and snacks, the phone. Except for my ever-present concern about the triplets reaching full term, I was pretty happy and carefree. A masseuse came twice a week, and a nurse also visited twice a week. My husband was very attentive and massaged me at least once a day. I enjoyed listening to Indian ragas, drinking my gallons of water!

My husband says I was in "the zone." I called it "incubator consciousness." I was content lying down, partly, I'm sure, because I was so uncomfortable being upright. The two hours I spent each day sitting up in our cooled-down hot tub gave me some variety and allowed digestion to take place. I am so grateful to have had a live-in helper.

In some sense, I felt like I was temporarily on vacation from life's normal responsibilities. All I had to do was grow those little babies inside of me. I was very happy.

Barry (33 years old)

At twenty-two, I was in a bad motorcycle accident. One afternoon, after just having gotten out of the shower, I decided to go up to a buddy's house. My helmet was in the house, and I thought no big deal, just three blocks and this way I can dry my hair. I proceeded up to his house; I knew the street really well— it was my neighborhood. As I was going around a blind turn, there was a truck parked right in the middle of the road. I could see that there was barely any space on either side of it, and I ended up crashing, sliding underneath the truck. I was pinned between the bike and the truck.

I sustained a head concussion, broken ribs, a broken cheekbone, and many bruises. I had severe lacerations on my leg from being pinned under the truck.

I was in the hospital in intensive care for three days, under general care for five days. I had 180 staples put in my leg. The brake peg was lodged in my calf. Luckily, there was no leg damage, but I just had to be stitched. I was released after a week and put on bed rest for the next month.

The television was my savior. I transferred my love of doing sports and being really fit to spectating sports via TV. My friends also made a huge difference in my bed rest. While my dad, with whom I lived, was no help at all, my friends were my lifeline. I could only manage to go to the bathroom on my own. My friends brought me fluids and food, and they checked in on me.

I never felt depressed. I was thankful to be alive. I spent a lot of my time talking on the phone with friends. And if I wasn't on the phone, I had a visitor. Ice cream made me feel better. I was in very good shape. I worried a little bit about just lying around, eating and drinking, but I knew once I healed, I would get back into great shape. I just kept a positive attitude and looked forward to getting back into my normal routine. I knew I wouldn't accomplish anything if I dwelled on the bad.

Sharon (66 years old)

Ten years ago, in the heat of the desert sun one afternoon, I fell into my wheelbarrow. I had tripped on the vines I was pruning. I fell hard, like no other fall I had ever taken. I was surprised at how awkwardly I had landed, and the next thing I knew, I was lying in the hospital in a dark room.

I had punctured my eyeballs on the vine's thorns. It was assumed I would be blind. I had surgery immediately and was left to recover for the next five months. Some of my therapy involved total stillness. The healing process was so fragile, any head motion would disturb an essential alignment that was trying to be retrieved.

I am a naturally meditative sort, and the stillness only strengthened my enjoyment of simply allowing time to pass. My children were grown and elsewhere, so my responsibilities were negligible. My husband was semiretired and very helpful with preparing and feeding me meals. I began losing weight with all of this change in lifestyle and eating patterns, and after about three weeks, we resorted to thick milk shakes in the heat of the afternoon. (My husband put on about eight pounds during this recovery period!).

Books on tape were my greatest source of joy and inspiration during the time of total stillness. My husband would often sit with me, rubbing my hands and forearms.

My role had always been to prepare and serve the meals and clean up around the house. Bob's commonsense responses to taking over almost everything in conjunction with his out-of-the-ordinary affection and concern was a drastic change. We both agree we felt a little like newlyweds, blessing each other's existence like there was no tomorrow. I strongly believe this change in our ways together hastened my healing. The experience took us beyond the physical and medical, to another world of spiritual unity. Our children, who came to visit many times, remarked on the dramatic change they observed in our recharged relationship!

My sight returned after six months of serious treatment. My

love of gardening has also returned, although it was almost a year from the time of the accident to the time when I returned to the garden. My husband gardens by my side almost daily. I believe this is less about being worried I will fall in the wheelbarrow again and more about enjoying our time together! My time of enforced quiet and stillness transformed our marriage.

APPENDIX A

Affirmations

The use of affirmations is a powerful tool in changing your consciousness and bringing a greater peace in your life. An affirmation is a positive thought held with conviction to produce a desired result. I used affirmations on a daily basis. They were my greatest source of strength and reinforcement of the goals I intended to accomplish on bed rest, most importantly a healthy delivery of my first child.

I have put together a collection of affirmations that are intended to encourage a hopeful frame of mind for your bed rest experience. If you find that you would rather use another kind of affirmation—a prayer, a poem, a quote or some other specific declaration, write it down and verbally state this positive thought every day. To affirm is to *make firm*—assertively to declare positive thoughts that will manifest positive results. Whatever affirmation(s) you choose, expect results!

I recommend verbalizing your affirmations and repeating them in private. Keep in mind, the use of affirmations requires a focus and attention that excludes outside distractions. You will want to approach this like you're proving to yourself that transformation will take place. As you say your affirmation, feel it and visualize it. Only thoughts with intense feeling bring results.

If you choose any of the passages below, highlight the one(s) that touch you. Read your selection(s) over and over, every day. If you give this exercise a chance, you will notice an improvement in your spirits. Affirmations also serve to reinforce important values for living. Open your mind and allow these affirmations to guide you to the limitless opportunities made available by your bed rest experience.

- I am living *every* moment to the fullest, on or off bed rest.
- I am here to learn.
- Right now, I accept myself as I am.
- I shall not agonize over this problem. I choose to greet life with courage, joy, and good humor.
- I respect the patterns of my unique life.
- I am capable of making a difference all around me, even when I am bedridden.
- I acknowledge my physical weakness and I feel strong.
- If it's to be, it's up to me. Anything!
- I watch my life's changing panorama with patience, acceptance, and good humor.
- I am flexible, resourceful, and open to new possibilities. I can adjust to life's changes, and I feel no need to resist. What is is what is now.
- I am living authentically, it matters not where I am.
- Movement is what creates life. To be still and still moving—this is everything!
- Stillness is what creates love.
- Bed rest is an opportunity for me right now. I am open to new insights. Like bamboo, I bend and grow, adjusting to the winds of change. I see within myself, take stock of my life, and set new goals.
- I am invigorated when I look at my life and know that I can accept bed rest and work with it.
- My life has many options. I am creative and resourceful.

I flow with the changes, seeing beyond the problems to solutions.

- 🌀 Laughter releases tension. Laughter heals all. I laugh on bed rest, too!
- 🌀 I trust this process without seeking to control it.
- 🌀 Wise people seek solutions; the ignorant only cast blame.
- 🌀 I can help myself and others so no one is lost. I will use my resources wisely so nothing is wasted.
- 🌀 I take many deep breaths and practice nonresistance.
- 🌀 My life is very peaceful now. I live with courage and compassion. I love and nurture myself. I do not criticize myself or others. I channel my energy into constructive outlets. I am loving and lovable. I accept greater peace in my world.
- 🌀 I have a reverence for life, a faith in the larger process. This faith sustains my experience, on or off bed rest. This faith affirms who I need to be at any moment. This faith affirms that I am on bed rest, and I will make the best of it.
- 🌀 Sustained by my faith, I do not fear change, nor do I surrender to adversity. I am courageous in being bedridden.
- 🌀 I am one with nature. In nature, everything is valuable, everything has its place. A rose, a daisy, a lark, a squirrel each manifests its potential differently, yet beautifully. On bed rest, I am still like a rock set on a hill. Like the rock, I move very little. I participate from my own place in life. The rock does not suffer from low self-esteem, nor do I.
- 🌀 Every day of bedrest is one in a succession of magical days. I am creating an experience that allows me to prosper on bed rest.
- 🌀 To make bed rest a meaningful existence, I am conscious of balancing giving and receiving. Right now, I communicate to myself and others what helps me and makes me feel special. I also ask what I can do for others.
- 🌀 As I think, so will I be.
- 🌀 My personal power is not aggressive, muscular, manipula-

tive, or authoritative power, but an inner power that comes from knowing I have all the resources I need to handle whatever happens in my life. When I feel my power, I shift from *appearing* strong to *feeling* strong. With the inner strength to face this challenge, I accept my bed rest experience on its own terms.

APPENDIX B

Self-help Bibliography

Recommended reading in alphabetical order by book title:

The 22 (Non-Negotiable) Laws of Wellness by Greg Anderson

All I Really Need to Know I Learned in Kindergarten: Uncommon Thoughts on Common Things by Robert Fulghum

The Aladin Factor by Jack Canfield and Mark Victor Hansen

The Almanac of Indispensable Information

Anatomy of an Illness by Norman Cousins

Anatomy of the Spirit: The Seven Stages of Power and Healing by Caroline Myss, Ph.D.

The Artist Way by Julia Cameron

Body Wisdom: An Easy-to-Use Handbook of Simple Exercises and Self-Massage Techniques for Busy People by Amiyo Ruhnke and Ananda Wurzburger

Chicken Soup for the Soul: 101 Stories to Open the Heart and Rekindle the Spirit by Jack Canfield and Mark Victor Hansen

Choose to Live Each Day Fully by Susan Smith Jones, Ph.D.

The Creative Spirit by Daniel Goleman, Ph.D.

Don't Panic, Taking Control of Anxiety Attacks by R. Reid Wilson, Ph.D.

Emotional Anatomy by Stanley Keleman

Emotional Intelligence by Daniel Goleman, Ph.D.

The Feeling Good Handbook by David Burns, M.D.

The Game of Life and How to Play It by Florence Scovel Shinon

A Guide for the Advanced Soul by Susan Hayward

The Healing Heart: Antidotes to Panic and Helplessness by Norman Cousins

The Health Effects of Attitudes, Emotions and Relationships by Brent Q. Hafen, Keith J. Karren, Kathryn J. Frandsen, N. Lee Smith

The Hidden Meaning of Illness by Bob Trowbridge, M.D.

Inner Simplicity by Elaine St. James

Life's Big Instruction Book by Carol Orsaf Madigan and Ann Elwood

Living Life on Purpose by Greg Anderson

Living the Mindful Life: A Handbook for Living in the Present Moment by Charles T. Tart

Love Is Letting Go of Fear by Gerald G. Jampolsky, M.D.

Man's Search for Meaning by Victor Frankl

The Meditative Mind by Daniel Goleman, Ph.D.

Mind as Healer, Mind as Slayer by Kenneth Pelletier

Minding the Body, Mending the Mind by Joan Borysenko, Ph.D.

The New Our Bodies Our Selves by The Boston Women's Health Book Collective

Peace Is Every Step by Thich Nhat Hanh

Pregnancy Bedrest by Susan H. Johnston and Deborah A. Kraut

Psychosomatics: How Your Emotions Can Damage Your Health by Howard R. and Martha E. Lewis

The Road Less Traveled by M. Scott Peck, M.D.

Simple Abundance by Sarah Ban Breathnach

Super Mind: The Ultimate Energy by Barbara B. Brown, Ph.D.

The Seven Spiritual Laws of Success by Deepak Chopra

Taming Your Mind: Enjoying, Experiencing, Discovering, Freeing, Understanding, Loving by Ken Keyes, Jr.

The Tao of Pooh by Benjamin Hoff

Total Wellness, Improve Your Health by Understanding the Body's Healing Systems by Joseph Pizzorno, M.D.

Touching: The Human Significance of the Skin by Ashley Montagu

Vital Lies, Simple Truths by Daniel Goleman, Ph.D.

Wake-Up Calls by Eric Allenbaugh

Wherever You Go, There You Are by Jon Kabat-Zinn, Ph.D.

Who Do You Think You Are? by Keith Harary, Ph.D. and Eileen Donahue, Ph.D.

You Can Heal Your Life by Louise L. Hay

You Can't Afford the Luxury of a Negative Thought by John Roger and Peter McWilliams

Your Body Believes Every Word You Say by Barbara Hoberman Levine

APPENDIX C

Who's Who at the Doctor's Office

When an unexpected and serious medical situation occurs, it is often easy to lose sight of who's who on your medical team. It is also common for physicians and their patients to experience poor communication, especially in the midst of crisis. Let's avoid this at all cost!

Here is a type of address book that will allow you to organize your medical care and log your questions and answers. When serious health issues are being confronted and emotions rise, it is difficult to think clearly, ask the appropriate questions, hear and understand the answers. And no matter how you may try to comprehend a doctor's prescription, it is a natural and healthy response to retain no more than a small bit at a time.

Never lose sight of the fact that it is *your right* to request time with your doctor and medical team. A planned telephone appointment will provide the time you need for your questions and the physicians' explanations. Here are some guidelines for getting the most out of your concerns and relationships:

1. Consider yourself an important member of your health-care team.

2. Approach your physician with respect and demand the same in return.
3. Prepare your concerns before your conversations and ask direct questions.
4. Be specific. Only you know exactly how you feel, where, when, etc.
5. Express your feelings in a direct but nonthreatening way.

You will feel empowered when you and your health-care providers work together to treat your medical problem. This kind of approach will not only enhance your care but can help to reduce stress and alleviate feelings of helplessness, hopelessness, incompetence, anger, and fear.

WHO'S WHO AT THE DOCTOR'S OFFICE

1. My Physician

Name:_____

Phone Number:_____

Pager (Get proper instructions):_____

Office Emergency Phone Number:_____

Hospital Phone Number:_____

My Doctor's Home Number (if appropriate):_____

Date—Question/Answer:

_____

_____

Date—Question/Answer:

_____

_____

Date—Question/Answer:

_____

_____

Date—Question/Answer:

_____

_____

_____

The important points my doctor has emphasized for optimal recovery:

_____

_____

_____

2. Back-up physician (partners, on-call backup team, etc.)

Name:_____

Phone Number:_____

Pager (Get proper instructions):_____

Office Emergency Phone Number:_____

Name:_____

Phone Number:_____

Pager (Get proper instructions):_____

Office Emergency Phone Number:_____

3. Other Medical Staff:

Nurses:

Name:_____

Phone Number:_____

Pager (Get proper instructions):_____

This person's unique role in my recovery:

_____

_____

Physical Therapist:

Name:_____

Phone Number:_____

Pager (Get proper instructions):_____

This person's unique role in my recovery:

_____

Other professionals (body work, lab technicians, pain program special-ist, pharmacist, etc.):

Name:_____

Phone Number:_____

Pager (Get proper instructions):_____

This person's unique role in my recovery:

_____

_____

_____

Name:_____

Phone Number:_____

Pager (Get proper instructions):_____

This person's unique role in my recovery:

_____

_____

_____

Name:_____

Phone Number:_____

Pager (Get proper instructions):_____

This person's unique role in my recovery:

_____

_____

_____

WHO'S WHO AT
THE DOCTOR'S
OFFICE

137

APPENDIX D

Important Phone Numbers

NAME_____

ADDRESS_____

CITY_____STATE_____ZIP_____

PHONE _____E-MAIL _____

NAME_____

ADDRESS_____

CITY_____STATE_____ZIP_____

PHONE _____E-MAIL _____

NAME_____

ADDRESS_____

CITY_____STATE_____ZIP_____

PHONE _____E-MAIL _____

NAME_____

ADDRESS_____

CITY_____STATE _____ZIP_____

PHONE _____E-MAIL _____

NAME_____

ADDRESS_____

CITY_____STATE _____ZIP_____

PHONE _____E-MAIL _____

NAME_____

ADDRESS_____

CITY_____STATE _____ZIP_____

PHONE _____E-MAIL _____

NAME_____

ADDRESS_____

CITY_____STATE _____ZIP_____

PHONE _____E-MAIL _____

NAME_____

ADDRESS_____

CITY_____STATE _____ZIP_____

PHONE _____E-MAIL _____

NAME_____

ADDRESS_____

Neighbors
and
Friends

CITY_____STATE _____ZIP_____

PHONE _____E-MAIL _____

NAME_____

ADDRESS_____

CITY_____STATE _____ZIP_____

PHONE _____E-MAIL _____

NAME_____

ADDRESS_____

CITY_____STATE _____ZIP_____

PHONE _____E-MAIL _____

NAME_____

ADDRESS_____

CITY_____STATE _____ZIP_____

PHONE _____E-MAIL _____

NAME_____

ADDRESS_____

CITY_____STATE _____ZIP_____

PHONE _____E-MAIL _____

NAME_____

ADDRESS_____

CITY_____STATE _____ZIP_____

PHONE _____E-MAIL _____

NAME_____

ADDRESS_____

CITY_____STATE _____ZIP_____

PHONE _____E-MAIL _____

NAME_____

ADDRESS_____

CITY_____STATE _____ZIP_____

PHONE _____E-MAIL _____

NAME_____

ADDRESS_____

CITY_____STATE _____ZIP_____

PHONE _____E-MAIL _____

NAME_____

ADDRESS_____

CITY_____STATE _____ZIP_____

PHONE _____E-MAIL _____

NAME_____

ADDRESS_____

CITY_____STATE _____ZIP_____

PHONE _____E-MAIL _____

NAME_____

ADDRESS_____

CITY_____STATE _____ZIP_____

PHONE _____E-MAIL _____

NAME_____

ADDRESS_____

CITY_____STATE _____ZIP_____

PHONE _____E-MAIL _____

NAME_____

ADDRESS_____

CITY_____STATE _____ZIP_____

PHONE _____E-MAIL _____

NAME_____

ADDRESS_____

CITY_____STATE _____ZIP_____

PHONE _____E-MAIL _____

NAME_____

ADDRESS_____

CITY_____STATE _____ZIP_____

PHONE _____E-MAIL _____

NAME_____

ADDRESS_____

CITY_____STATE _____ZIP_____

PHONE _____E-MAIL _____

Medical Information

NAME_____

ADDRESS_____

CITY_____STATE _____ZIP_____

PHONE _____E-MAIL _____

NAME_____

ADDRESS_____

CITY_____STATE _____ZIP_____

PHONE _____E-MAIL _____

NAME_____

ADDRESS_____

CITY_____STATE_____ZIP_____

PHONE_____E-MAIL_____

~~~~~~

NAME_____

ADDRESS_____

CITY_____STATE_____ZIP_____

PHONE_____E-MAIL_____

~~~~~~

NAME_____

ADDRESS_____

CITY_____STATE_____ZIP_____

PHONE_____E-MAIL_____

~~~~~~

NAME_____

ADDRESS_____

CITY_____STATE_____ZIP_____

PHONE_____E-MAIL_____

~~~~~~

NAME_____

ADDRESS_____

CITY_____STATE_____ZIP_____

PHONE _____E-MAIL _____

NAME_____

ADDRESS_____

CITY_____STATE_____ZIP_____

PHONE _____E-MAIL _____

Physical
Therapy/
Bodywork

NAME_____

ADDRESS_____

CITY_____STATE_____ZIP_____

PHONE _____E-MAIL _____

NAME_____

ADDRESS_____

CITY_____STATE_____ZIP_____

PHONE _____E-MAIL _____

NAME_____

ADDRESS_____

CITY_____STATE _____ZIP_____

PHONE _____E-MAIL _____

NAME_____

ADDRESS_____

CITY_____STATE _____ZIP_____

PHONE _____E-MAIL _____

NAME_____

ADDRESS_____

CITY_____STATE _____ZIP_____

PHONE _____E-MAIL _____

NAME_____

ADDRESS_____

CITY_____STATE _____ZIP_____

PHONE _____E-MAIL _____

Physical
Therapy/
Bodywor

NAME_____

ADDRESS_____

CITY_____STATE _____ZIP_____

PHONE _____E-MAIL _____

NAME_____

ADDRESS_____

CITY_____STATE _____ZIP_____

PHONE _____E-MAIL _____

NAME_____

ADDRESS_____

CITY_____STATE _____ZIP_____

PHONE _____E-MAIL _____

NAME_____

ADDRESS_____

CITY_____STATE _____ZIP_____

PHONE _____E-MAIL _____

Money
Matters

NAME_____

ADDRESS_____

CITY_____STATE _____ZIP_____

PHONE _____E-MAIL _____

NAME_____

ADDRESS_____

CITY_____STATE _____ZIP_____

PHONE _____E-MAIL _____

NAME_____

ADDRESS_____

CITY_____STATE _____ZIP_____

PHONE _____E-MAIL _____

NAME_____

ADDRESS_____

CITY_____STATE _____ZIP_____

PHONE _____E-MAIL _____

NAME_____

ADDRESS_____

CITY_____STATE _____ZIP_____

PHONE _____E-MAIL _____

NAME_____

ADDRESS_____

CITY_____STATE _____ZIP_____

PHONE _____E-MAIL _____

NAME_____

ADDRESS_____

CITY_____STATE _____ZIP_____

PHONE _____E-MAIL _____

NAME_____

ADDRESS_____

CITY_____STATE _____ZIP_____

PHONE _____E-MAIL _____

NAME_____

ADDRESS_____

CITY_____STATE _____ZIP_____

PHONE _____E-MAIL _____

❧❧❧❧❧❧❧❧❧❧❧❧❧❧❧❧❧❧❧❧❧❧❧❧❧❧❧

NAME_____

ADDRESS_____

CITY_____STATE _____ZIP_____

PHONE _____E-MAIL _____

❧❧❧❧❧❧❧❧❧❧❧❧❧❧❧❧❧❧❧❧❧❧❧❧❧❧❧

NAME_____

ADDRESS_____

CITY_____STATE _____ZIP_____

PHONE _____E-MAIL _____

❧❧❧❧❧❧❧❧❧❧❧❧❧❧❧❧❧❧❧❧❧❧❧❧❧❧❧

NAME_____

ADDRESS_____

CITY_____STATE _____ZIP_____

PHONE _____E-MAIL _____

❧❧❧❧❧❧❧❧❧❧❧❧❧❧❧❧❧❧❧❧❧❧❧❧❧❧❧

NAME_____

ADDRESS_____

CITY_____STATE_____ZIP_____

PHONE_____E-MAIL_____

NAME_____

ADDRESS_____

CITY_____STATE_____ZIP_____

PHONE_____E-MAIL_____

NAME_____

ADDRESS_____

CITY_____STATE_____ZIP_____

PHONE_____E-MAIL_____

NAME_____

ADDRESS_____

CITY_____STATE_____ZIP_____

PHONE_____E-MAIL_____

NAME_____

ADDRESS_____

CITY_____STATE _____ZIP_____

PHONE _____E-MAIL _____

NAME_____

ADDRESS_____

CITY_____STATE _____ZIP_____

PHONE _____E-MAIL _____

NAME_____

ADDRESS_____

CITY_____STATE _____ZIP_____

PHONE _____E-MAIL _____

NAME_____

ADDRESS_____

CITY_____STATE _____ZIP_____

PHONE _____E-MAIL _____

NAME_____

ADDRESS_____

CITY_____STATE _____ZIP_____

PHONE _____E-MAIL _____

NAME_____

ADDRESS_____

CITY_____STATE _____ZIP_____

PHONE _____E-MAIL _____

NAME_____

ADDRESS_____

CITY_____STATE _____ZIP_____

PHONE _____E-MAIL _____

NAME_____

ADDRESS_____

CITY_____STATE _____ZIP_____

PHONE _____E-MAIL _____

NAME_____

ADDRESS_____

CITY_____STATE _____ZIP_____

PHONE _____E-MAIL _____

NAME_____

ADDRESS_____

CITY_____STATE _____ZIP_____

PHONE _____E-MAIL _____

NAME_____

ADDRESS_____

CITY_____STATE _____ZIP_____

PHONE _____E-MAIL _____

NAME_____

ADDRESS_____

CITY_____STATE _____ZIP_____

PHONE _____E-MAIL _____

NAME_____

ADDRESS_____

CITY_____STATE _____ZIP_____

PHONE _____E-MAIL _____

NAME_____

ADDRESS_____

CITY_____STATE _____ZIP_____

PHONE _____E-MAIL _____

NAME_____

ADDRESS_____

CITY_____STATE _____ZIP_____

PHONE _____E-MAIL _____

NAME_____

ADDRESS_____

CITY_____STATE _____ZIP_____

PHONE _____E-MAIL _____

NAME_____

ADDRESS_____

CITY_____STATE _____ZIP_____

PHONE _____E-MAIL _____

NAME_____

ADDRESS_____

CITY_____STATE _____ZIP_____

PHONE _____E-MAIL _____

NAME_____

ADDRESS_____

CITY_____STATE _____ZIP_____

PHONE _____E-MAIL _____

NAME_____

ADDRESS_____

CITY_____STATE _____ZIP_____

PHONE _____E-MAIL _____

Kids'
Contacts

NAME_____

ADDRESS_____

CITY_____STATE _____ZIP_____

PHONE _____E-MAIL _____

NAME_____

ADDRESS_____

CITY_____STATE _____ZIP_____

PHONE _____E-MAIL _____

NAME_____

ADDRESS_____

CITY_____STATE _____ZIP_____

PHONE _____E-MAIL _____

NAME_____

ADDRESS_____

CITY_____STATE _____ZIP_____

PHONE _____E-MAIL _____

Personal
Project
Supplies

NAME_____

ADDRESS_____

CITY_____STATE _____ZIP_____

PHONE _____E-MAIL _____

NAME_____

ADDRESS_____

CITY_____STATE _____ZIP_____

PHONE _____E-MAIL _____

NAME_____

ADDRESS_____

CITY_____STATE _____ZIP_____

PHONE _____E-MAIL _____

NAME_____

ADDRESS_____

CITY_____STATE _____ZIP_____

PHONE _____E-MAIL _____

Personal
Project
Supplies

APPENDIX E

Home Services and Supply Sources

In your search to access the many different services that will assist you in making the most of your bed rest experience, begin by tapping into local resource centers. Networking is the name of the game on bed rest. You may not meet your needs the first time you try to find a piece of equipment, medical aid, house-cleaner, or physical therapist, but chances are every telephone call you make will bring you closer to your goal. Calling around will allow you to locate what you need, compare supplies, quality of equipment, pricing, rental and lease options, and delivery services.

When you reach someone who has information and can potentially fulfill your request, always explain your bed rest condition and be very specific about your limitations. Since it is impossible for *The Bed Rest Survival Guide* to supply specific resources for every geographical location in the United States, the following guidelines are recommended to begin networking:

1. telephone the central hospital or medical facility in your area
2. telephone the main library in your vicinity

3. look up Home Health Services in the Yellow Pages (also try under Health, Rehabilitation, Sports Medicine, Physical Therapy, Disability, Equipment, Medical Equipment, Back)
4. inquire at a local athletic club or spa
5. word of mouth—never hesitate to ask any questions about how to find anything from relatives, friends, co-workers

SUPPLIES AND SERVICES

Durable medical equipment:

For temporary bed rest, local sources are usually the most convenient and economical.

- Yellow Pages under Home Health Care or Medical Equipment
- Local hospital or hospice
- Pharmacies
- Large chain store, e.g. Payless, Thrifty, Costco, etc.
- Medical supply store
- Sports medicine clinic
- Urgent care center
- Physical Therapy Center
- Apria 1-800-APRIA-88
- Lincare 1-800-260-0124
- Home Healthcare Services 1-800-406-6650
- Visiting Nurses Association of America (Headquarters) 1-303-753-0218

You may also find useful supplies via mail-order catalogs. I suggest you use the toll free numbers and request a catalog from each of the following services. You never know—you may see something that introduces new possibilities for your bed rest experience!

Catalogs:

- Mountainville House Calls 1-800-460-7282
- Self Care 1-800-345-3371
- BackSaver 1-800-251-2225
- Levenger 1-800-544-0880
- Living Arts 1-800-254-8464
- Hold Everything 1-800-421-2264
- Hands-On Health Care Catalog 1-800-442-2232
- Anderson Bedroom Organizer 1-800-782-4825
- Home Office 1-800-869-6000
- The Magellan Group's Tools for Living 1-800-644-8100 Ext. US291

Meal providers:

- Home Catering Companies, e.g. Meals on Wheels. "Extended Family" is a company that delivers a week's worth of nutritionally balanced, home-cooked meals anywhere in the continental U.S. Prices start at approximately $55 for a week of dinners for one. Shipping is extra. For a free catalog and menu, call 800-235-7070.
- Local Restaurant Delivery
- Visiting Nurses Association of America (Headquarters) 1-303-753-0218

Medical aids and personal assistance:

- Ask your doctor
- Visiting Nurses Association of America (Headquarters) 1-303-753-0218
- Sidelines National Support 1-714-497-2265. This group has over thirty chapters around the country and support coverage in every state. It matches a woman on pregnancy bed rest with a peer counselor who has been through a similar experience. For educational matierals, call 1-714-651-8673.
- Home Healthcare Services 1-800-406-6650

Housecleaning:

- Network with neighbors and friends
- Bulletin boards at local centers i.e. athletic clubs, neighborhood grocery, schools
- Community newspaper
- Yellow Pages
- Local high school job counselor

Personal organizer:

- It makes an enormous difference to have someone come into your home once a week or once a month to organize the piles that inevitably develop in a household when someone is bedridden. This person is not necessarily a professional. It is someone who is usually known through the community with excellent organizational skills. This person can be your mother, aunt, sister, brother! When hired, it is essential that this person understand their role as an organizer and not someone who arbitrarily throws things out. This person must be able to follow instructions so that papers are well managed: reviewed, organized, categorized, and cleaned. The final phase of this kind of work should involve clear communication back to you so that you are aware of the location of important personal and household material.

Handyperson:

If there is no one around to take care of changing lightbulbs, installing bed rest equipment, plumbing problems, childproofing in the case of single parenting, etc., a maintenance professional is the answer. How to find one?

- Word of mouth
- Local hardware-store referral
- Local newspaper/classified section
- Yellow Pages under Home, Maintenance, Handy
- Bulletin board at neighborhood grocery, laundromat, etc.

Bookkeeper/accountant:

- A local accounting firm may have interns who can take over bill paying
- The local newspaper almost always has classified ads for home bookkeepers
- A friend
- Your partner

Entertainment:

Laughing and feeling good is integral to the healing process. Depending on what kind of person you are and your medical problem, the following may be more impactful than a nurse's aide:

- Home video delivery
- Caterers
- Beautician—hair and face
- Body work
- Puppet shows
- Magic shows
- Balloons
- Cooking lessons (you stay on a cot while the instructor demonstrates)
- Music lessons
- Voice lessons
- Screenplays for your family and/or friends to perform

Acknowledgments

It has been a great source of fulfillment to write a book that has the potential to uplift those who find themselves in a situation that at first seems intolerable. As other writers know, it's a long process, and one rarely does it alone. In every corner of my life, there was someone offering something specific to this project. In the very early stages, at a time when I didn't know whether to continue my high-tech marketing career or to focus exclusively on writing the book, my friend, Amy Slater, pushed for me to *go for the book.* I am so grateful for this and other assertive friends who weren't afraid to speak up and provide the necessary pushes.

I would like to express my love and gratitude to the following people:

Our extraordinary friend, Ursula Flache, and her husband, Volker, who always took an interest and reached out to help with our children. Another friend, Trisha Schaller, after having read the first draft of the first chapter, immediately proposed I write from my own experience rather than in the third person. This important shift opened up an infinitely more rewarding writing experience and has drawn me very close to every reader.

Jeffrey Abrahams consulted me on editing and publishing protocol. His intelligence and open heart lit the way not only for me but the many people who will read this book.

Margaret Livingston and Lynne Bosche found many extra hours in their already overcommitted lives to critique and edit chapter sections. Each of their contributions significantly shaped the end result of this book.

My two culinary friends, Julie Hamilton and Patty Scott, consulted on the Smart and Savory Picnics chapter and graciously offered detailed suggestions and trade secrets. My swimming friends, Morris and Audrey Weiss, Helen Nestor, Helene Zeiger, Harvey Bailey, Betsy Cohen, and Karin Zeldin each put their own creative stamp on this book.

My long-distance friends Julie Childs, Pam Smilow, and Andrea Eschen nourished me with the purest love and encouragement friendship knows. Each also provided critique and connections to others who have experienced bed rest.

Owen Mulholland's, Richard Cowan's, and Sue Levin's professionalism provided me with enhanced confidence at various junctures. Edward Farmer's spriritual guidance and forthright confidence-building made a difference in the completion of this project. Christine and Doug Cram designed and produced a mockup of the book that I believe enchanted not only my agent but my publisher.

I am so appreciative of the many testimonial writers whose experiences have been incorporated throughout the text. Each veteran bedrester enthusiastically volunteered his or her story as a way to reach out and have an impact on all of the readers. The time, effort, and passion to share themselves has contributed significantly to the quality of the book. And without the help from various friends who volunteered to pass out my questionnaires and surveys to anyone they knew or had heard about on bed rest, much of the book's essence would be missing. Special thanks to Felicia Lu, M.D. and John Citron, M.D., whose friendship was born out of the shared experience of bed rest and their desire to see this book published.

Hallie Beacham, M.D., M.P.H., my OB-Gyn and longtime friend, provided immeasurable validation, support, and material.

My parents and my sisters stood behind my determination and wanted the best for this book. My mother went to great efforts to provide medical advice and connections to bed rest veterans. My in-laws, Deirdrellen and Carrell Peterson, provided the kind of loving assistance that made it possible for me to manage my family life and write this book.

Words cannot properly describe the love and appreciation I have for my immediate family, Dick, Hilary, and Foreste. We four know what a huge family stretch it has been to make this book a reality. My husband's love of music went by the wayside every car trip we took. Instead, for the last year, he listened to every word of every sentence and contributed greatly to the clarity of every chapter. Thousands of my telephone interruptions at his work were met with a kind, positive response and keen ear to help fix many writing obstacles. I never knew a partner could be so patient and deeply committed. My daughters, Hilary and Foreste, energize me and encourage me every day to reach for the stars. My family has given this book its radiant blessings.

ACKNOWLEDGMENT.

165